Just in time, this volume addresses a gap in the resurging literature on existential–humanistic psychotherapy: the scarcity of guidebooks elucidating existential–humanistic assessment and case formulation. Drawing on an impressive array of quantitative and qualitative research, the authors have managed to put together a practical and philosophically faithful framework that can be readily accessed by both graduate-level trainees and seasoned professionals. In that light I am thrilled to recommend this book as a gateway to an existential–humanistic revival, both in the classroom and the clinic.

–KIRK J. SCHNEIDER, PhD, EDITOR OF *EXISTENTIAL-INTEGRATIVE PSYCHOTHERAPY: GUIDEPOSTS TO THE CORE OF PRACTICE*; COAUTHOR OF *EXISTENTIAL-HUMANISTIC THERAPY, THIRD EDITION*; AND COAUTHOR OF *THE PSYCHOLOGY OF EXISTENCE: AN INTEGRATIVE, CLINICAL PERSPECTIVE*

Hoffman and Cleare-Hoffman provide an innovative framework for contemporary existential–humanistic case formulation with a liberatory dimension. Drawing on rich clinical illustrations, this unique volume centers sociocultural context in existential–humanistic theory and translates theory to moment-to-moment interactions between client and therapist. It is a must-read volume for practitioners, educators, and researchers interested in a nuanced and holistic understanding of therapeutic process.

–PRATYUSHA TUMMALA-NARRA, PhD, DEPARTMENT OF COUNSELING, DEVELOPMENTAL AND EDUCATIONAL PSYCHOLOGY, BOSTON COLLEGE, CHESTNUT HILL, MA

I was thrilled to read this book! It makes clear why existential–humanistic (EH) approaches are central to any social justice-oriented therapy. The authors provide a foundation of respect in which therapy is tailored to clients within their own cultural contexts and experiences. Reading this book is even better than being able to peer into the sessions of eminent therapists, because you can both see their interventions and hear their thoughts on how best to empower and support clients. Students will love that the framing of the book is centered on focused case examples, allowing for a rich clinical understanding of how EH conceptualization develops across time when working with a client. I have long admired the leadership and expertise that these authors bring to existential–humanistic psychotherapy and appreciate the sensitivity they bring to each page. Students will learn how to apply interventions, but they will learn so much more as well. The text supports them to become truly responsive therapists in the service of their clients.

–HEIDI M. LEVITT, PhD, PROFESSOR, DEPARTMENT OF PSYCHOLOGY, UNIVERSITY OF MASSACHUSETTS BOSTON

Case Formulation in Existential–Humanistic Therapy is a landmark text that fills an enormous gap in the literature. Often my students complain that much of the current literature in existential and humanistic therapy digs deep into the philosophical foundations of the practice, but they find it difficult to translate the theory into practice. This book changes the game. Experienced professional therapists and graduate students will find this book to be refreshingly clear and pragmatic in its focus. This book is essential reading for therapists who wish to learn how to navigate the task of approaching case formulation and treatment planning within an existential–humanistic framework.

—**BRENT DEAN ROBBINS, PhD,** PROFESSOR OF PSYCHOLOGY,
POINT PARK UNIVERSITY, PITTSBURGH, PA

All practitioners and learners of existential–humanistic (EH) therapy are likely to rejoice at the release of this book. It provides the type of loose structure that will help contain the anxious unknowing of trainees, the unarticulated knowing of professors and supervisors, and the floundering frustrations of established clinicians alike—all while giving EH practitioners the freedom to maintain their unique integrative styles. Any course that teaches the theory and practice of existential and humanistic therapies would benefit greatly from this book.

—**BRIAN S. HANNA, PsyD,** LICENSED CLINICAL PSYCHOLOGIST,
HANNA PSYCHOLOGICAL SERVICES, PARK RIDGE, IL

This book fills a critical void for those seeking case conceptualization from an existential–humanistic orientation. Its approach to case formulation is practical and flexible, and it emphasizes collaboration with clients. It will be essential reading for psychotherapists, diagnostic clinicians, as well as medical doctors and researchers (e.g., of therapeutic outcome studies) and will be invaluable to both seasoned practitioners and students in training.

—**DAN HOCOY, PhD,** LICENSED CLINICAL PSYCHOLOGIST; CONSULTING EDITOR,
THE HUMANISTIC PSYCHOLOGIST; AND PRESIDENT, GODDARD COLLEGE, PLAINFIELD, VT

CASE FORMULATION IN

EXISTENTIAL-HUMANISTIC THERAPY

CASE FORMULATION IN
EXISTENTIAL-HUMANISTIC THERAPY

LOUIS HOFFMAN &
HEATHERLYN P.
CLEARE-HOFFMAN

 AMERICAN PSYCHOLOGICAL ASSOCIATION

Published by
American Psychological Association
750 First Street, NE
Washington, DC 20002
https://www.apa.org

Order Department
https://www.apa.org/pubs/books
order@apa.org

Typeset in Meridien and Ortodoxa by Circle Graphics, Inc., Reisterstown, MD

Printer: Gasch Printing, Odenton, MD
Cover Designer: Mark Karis

Library of Congress Cataloging-in-Publication Data

Names: Hoffman, Louis, author. | Cleare-Hoffman, Heatherlyn, author.
Title: Case formulation in existential-humanistic therapy / by Louis
    Hoffman & Heatherlyn P. Cleare-Hoffman.
Description: Washington, DC : American Psychological Association, [2025] |
    Includes bibliographical references and index.
Identifiers: LCCN 2024051224 (print) | LCCN 2024051225 (ebook) | ISBN
    9781433842948 (paperback) | ISBN 9781433842955 (ebook)
Subjects: LCSH: Experiential psychotherapy. | Humanistic psychology.
Classification: LCC RC489.E96 H64 2025 (print) | LCC RC489.E96 (ebook) |
    DDC 616.89/14--dc23/eng/20250307
LC record available at https://lccn.loc.gov/2024051224
LC ebook record available at https://lccn.loc.gov/2024051225

https://doi.org/10.1037/0000464-000

Printed in the United States of America

10 9 8 7 6 5 4 3 2 1

To our sons, Lakoda, Lukaya, and Lyon.

CONTENTS

Acknowledgments ix

**Introduction: A Phenomenological and Liberatory Approach
to Case Formulation** **3**

1. **A Framework for Existential-Humanistic Case Formulation** **13**

2. **Existential-Humanistic Treatment Approaches: Identifying
   and Mapping Interventions** **41**

3. **Case Example Introduction: Rasheeda** **63**

4. **Brief Holistic Client Narrative** **87**

5. **Concern or Problem Identification** **93**

6. **Theoretical Aspects of the Case Formulation** **105**

7. **Treatment Planning** **147**

8. **Support for Treatment Approaches, Stances, and/or
   Techniques** **157**

9. **Additional Case Illustrations of Existential-Humanistic
   Case Formulation** **165**

**Epilogue: Concluding Thoughts on Existential-Humanistic
Therapy Case Formulation** **205**

Appendix A: Existential–Humanistic Case Formulation 207
Appendix B: Recommended Reading for Existential–Humanistic Theory
   and Psychotherapy 219
References 225
Index 237
About the Authors 243

ACKNOWLEDGMENTS

The encouragement of several people was important in this book coming to fruition. Michael Moats regularly encouraged Louis to make this project a priority. Several individuals reviewed chapters of this book and provided feedback, including Kirk Schneider, Shawn Rubin, Theopia Jackson, Michael Moats, Brittany Varisco, and Jeff Singer. Discussions with Terri Davis and Sabah Islam also led to specific refinements.

As part of the original design of developing this approach to case formulation and treatment planning, we taught this approach in several settings to help refine it. First, Louis presented this approach in China through the International Institute for Existential Psychology in the summer of 2018. The discussions led to refinements of the approach. The Existential and Humanistic Theory and Therapy class at the University of Denver, Winter 2020, was the first class to use an earlier version of the case formulation template. Along with students in this class doing an impressive job with the case formulations, class discussions were instrumental in the most significant advancements of this approach since the original version. It has subsequently been used at the University of Denver in 2021, 2022, 2023, and 2024. While there were fewer refinements as the model solidified, the continued opportunities to teach the model in training settings influenced the development of this book.

Ed Meidenbauer contacted me (Louis) in 2018 to see if I had any ideas for projects with American Psychological Association (APA) Videos or APA Books. I met with Ed and Susan Reynolds shortly after this and pitched the idea for a two-volume book series on existential–humanistic case formulation and evidence-based foundations of existential–humanistic therapy. Ed suggested that we could do a video with these books. When I first proposed these projects, I was still deep in commitments that I was behind on due to a heavy academic load. I appreciate that Ed and Susan continued to stay in contact about these projects. The initial proposals were delayed, and then the writing of the book was delayed due to a shoulder injury and surgery that made typing difficult for some time, as well as taking on the *APA Handbook of Humanistic and Existential Psychology*. Ed and Susan's patience and encouragement were meaningful and instrumental in seeing this book, as well as the video and companion volume, come to fruition.

While finishing this book, I (Louis) filmed a related video, *Existential–Humanistic Case Formulation*, with APA Videos. The entire team at APA Books and Videos that I worked with, especially Susan, Ed, and Lisa Osorio, is greatly appreciated and deserves special acknowledgment. Particularly instrumental was Theopia Jackson, who interviewed me following the recording of the session with the client. Theopia's expert consultation about the video helped further our thinking about case formulation.

I (Louis) would like to thank the Rocky Mountain Humanistic Counseling and Psychotherapy Association's board, who have provided support and encouragement throughout the writing process. I would particularly like to thank Nathaniel Granger Jr., H. Luis Vargas, Francis Kaklauskas, and Ian Wickramasekera II for their support and for being part of our annual writing retreat, an important space for writing and thinking through projects. Last, I would like to thank the University of Denver's (DU) Graduate School of Psychology. The opportunity to teach and supervise at DU has played a significant role in how the final product developed over time.

I (Heatherlyn) express my deepest gratitude to Chrissy Roth and Shea Voelker, two of my best friends, for their continued support. They have supported me whenever I needed it and continue to believe in me even when I don't believe in myself. For that, I am eternally grateful.

CASE FORMULATION IN

EXISTENTIAL-
HUMANISTIC
THERAPY

Introduction

A Phenomenological and Liberatory Approach to Case Formulation

Existential–humanistic (EH) therapists historically eschewed case formulation on a philosophical basis, raising concerns about how this process objectifies and pathologizes clients, negatively impacts the therapy process, and limits the scope of treatment. In addition, EH therapists are concerned that the process is hierarchical rather than collaborative, which increases the power differential between client and therapist. These concerns, along with other critiques of case formulation, make it important to ask at the outset of this project, "Why develop an existential–humanistic approach to case formulation?" Over the past 20 years, we have worked in various graduate programs in psychology and training sites and trained many students in EH therapy, including at a training clinic we founded in Colorado Springs, as well as other settings and graduate programs in psychology. This experience made it apparent that many students encountered problems in their graduate programs and training sites when using an EH approach. This was partly due to the growing monoculture in psychology, resulting in few faculty members and supervisors being well-versed in EH psychology (see Levy & Anderson, 2013). However, there was more to it.

One challenge emerged when students approached their comprehensive evaluations in graduate school. Being required to complete a case formulation remains a common approach to comprehensive examinations in many graduate programs. Because there were no models for doing these from an EH perspective, students wanting to use this approach on their exams had to create their own approach. While some of these were well thought out and

---

https://doi.org/10.1037/0000464-001
Case Formulation in Existential–Humanistic Therapy, by L. Hoffman and H. P. Cleare-Hoffman

implemented, faculty members often struggled to know how to evaluate them. At other times, students who were just learning the approach struggled to develop a well-grounded approach to EH case formulation. The result was that many good students, who were also good therapists, failed their exams. Over time, as word spread about the challenges their peers faced, other students abandoned trying to use EH case formulations.

In training contexts, many students are similarly required to do a case formulation, frequently encountering similar problems. Students have been told that this is not a stand-alone therapy, there is insufficient structure for case formulations, and there is insufficient evidence to support the efficacy or effectiveness of EH therapy. Some of this is understandable. Yalom (1980), who is sometimes associated with EH therapy, advocated that it is not a stand-alone approach. However, we maintain that while Yalom shares many similarities with EH therapy, his approach is better understood as his own existential therapy that has some commonalities with EH therapy. Also, there have been limited direct outcome studies on EH therapy (see Bland, 2026). The limited research is partly due to the lack of a guide for EH therapy. The development of an EH approach to case formulation provides a foundation for conducting outcome research.

Students interested in EH therapy often report struggles with learning how to implement EH therapy, including how to track themes, when to implement particular treatment strategies, and how to track progress. The lack of structure often creates anxiety for these students. The EH case formulation approach brings a flexible structure that is useful for students learning this approach. While, at times, some of the nuance is lost in the structure, the structure can be an important part of a development process of learning EH therapy. As students grow in their theoretical and practical understanding of EH therapy, they will be better able to address aspects of the nuance and flexibility that may be less evident in earlier stages of professional development.

It is not only students who are challenged by the lack of an EH approach to case formulation. This has contributed to challenges for EH therapists working with insurance reimbursement and working in some mental health settings. In large part, this, again, is due to the perception of the lack of research and difficulty demonstrating the effectiveness of EH therapy. In addition to providing a foundation for conducting outcome research, a model for case formulation could provide a method for demonstrating the effectiveness of EH therapy based on current research (see Hoffman & Lac, 2025).

Licensed EH therapists often encounter challenges in some agency settings and in working with insurance companies because of the lack of a more structured model for case formulation, including problem identification and treatment planning. Similarly, because many EH therapists prefer to avoid diagnosis, case formulation can be used as an alternative to diagnosis in some settings (Johnstone, 2018). Developing an EH case formulation approach may help EH therapists achieve greater freedom in implementing this approach to therapy.

These struggles of our students and colleagues were the inspiration for creating an approach to EH case formulation and writing this book. EH case formulation, therefore, has practical utility for students, licensed therapists, and researchers in guiding the therapeutic process and advocating for a place for EH therapy in many settings that are often resistant to this approach. We hope *Case Formulation in Existential–Humanistic Therapy* will fill an important void and serve as a foundation for future research and scholarship on EH therapy.

EXISTENTIAL–HUMANISTIC CASE FORMULATION AND THERAPY DEVELOPMENT

Becoming an EH therapist is not easy (see Falk & Hoffman, 2022). In part, this is because becoming an EH therapist is primarily about the development of the person of the therapist, particularly the relational therapeutic qualities, instead of learning specific techniques or structured treatment strategies. In addition, it is largely a techniqueless approach (Hoffman, 2019c). For students and early career therapists learning this approach, it can be intimidating because it lacks the structure that other approaches rely on. While there are therapeutic advantages to this, it also can make it more difficult to learn.

While the approach to case formulation articulated in this book is not intended to change the therapeutic approach, it does provide a degree of structure that may aid individuals trying to learn EH therapy. We hope this makes it less intimidating to learn, even if some aspects of the complexity of EH therapy are more difficult to highlight within the structure. These can be addressed in other areas of training, such as clinical supervision. The formulation process helps therapists track themes emerging in therapy, allowing for greater consideration about how to clarify and work with these themes therapeutically. It can also help track therapeutic progress on specific issues. As many therapists become more established, they rely on the structure less because the process has become more natural and ingrained. Therefore, we designed this approach to have a structure for case formulation and a structure for learning this approach to therapy that, over time, can be relied on less.

WHO THIS BOOK IS FOR

This book is designed primarily for students with some familiarity with EH therapy, clinical supervisors, and professors in academic settings who are teaching EH therapy or grading comprehensive examinations of EH case formulations. It also has utility for researchers and licensed professionals. For researchers, the case formulation approach provides a basic structure that can be used for conducting outcome research on EH therapy. For licensed therapists, the approach can help advance their therapy skills, provide ways for tracking progress on themes, and advocate for the appropriateness of EH therapy in certain settings and with insurance companies. We hope that each therapist's use of this will evolve over time. As students, completing a case formulation aids in learning how to do EH therapy and can guide the treatment process over time, including helping to see how EH therapy evolves over the course of treatment. However, clinicians will likely gradually use more abbreviated versions of this form and adapt it to their needs. After completing several of these, this may become more of an implicit process with therapists instead of writing out a full case formulation with each client they see.

While the primary focus is on EH students, practitioners, and researchers, it may also be useful to medical doctors, psychiatric nurse practitioners, agency supervisors and administrators, and insurance companies. This approach to case formulation can help these individuals recognize the utility of an EH approach, including when referrals to EH therapists are appropriate.

DEVELOPMENT OF THE APPROACH

The process of developing an EH approach to case formulation began with research. In 2017, we conducted a research study on the primary influences on EH therapy and factors that EH therapists felt were important to consider in case formulation (Cleare-Hoffman & Hoffman, 2017; Hoffman & Cleare-Hoffman, 2017a). Research on the primary influences was important in clarifying seminal authors and works, which is used in Chapter 2 to determine the texts included to identify and clarify EH interventions. The results overall were not surprising, with Rollo May being identified as the primary influence on EH theory and James F. T. Bugental being the primary influence on therapy applications (Cleare-Hoffman & Hoffman, 2017). Other influences included Kirk Schneider, Irvin Yalom, Viktor Frankl, Carl Rogers, R. D. Laing, Myrtle Heery, David Elkins, Mick Cooper, Orah Krug, Fritz Perls, Erik Craig, and Louis Hoffman. Some of these figures do not identify as EH therapists but are in related branches, such as humanistic psychology and daseinsanalysis.

The second paper from this research focused on the components identified to be included in EH case formulation (Hoffman & Cleare-Hoffman, 2017b; see also Chapter 2, this volume), resulting in the initial case formulation template. The findings were presented as poster presentations, which allowed for conversations about the approach. Minor revisions were made from the feedback. Later that year, a paper was presented focusing on multicultural considerations of EH case formulation (Hoffman & Cleare-Hoffman, 2017b), followed by presentations in 2018 and 2019 (Cleare-Hoffman & Hoffman, 2018; Hoffman, 2019a; Hoffman & Cleare-Hoffman, 2018a, 2018b). In addition, one of us (Louis) began teaching about the approach through the International Institute of Existential–Humanistic Therapy in China and the University of Denver. These further presentations and teaching of the model resulted in more minor changes. Feedback from Terri Davis, the program director at the University of Denver's PsyD program at the time, and Sabah Islam, a student who learned this approach in class, also resulted in modifications.

In summary, the initial formulations were based on research and reviews of seminal texts combined with our experience as EH practitioners. Feedback from professional presentations and students learning this approach led to several minor revisions, resulting in the current version presented in this book and the template developed for EH case formulation (see Appendix A).

CAN CASE FORMULATION HAVE A LIBERATORY FRAMEWORK?

An argument could be made that case formulation tends to be colonizing. Most approaches to case formulation interpret the client primarily through theory and, at times, research. Both the theory and research emerged largely from psychological theory and research reflecting the dominant culture's values. In the history of psychology, this means that White Eurocentric theory and research provided the foundation for the frames through which therapists conceptualize, diagnose, and understand their clients.

This is partially due to what Pablo Freire (1970/2009) described as a banking approach to education applied to psychology. Banking models of education focus on the accumulation of knowledge that has been deemed the "right" knowledge by the "elites" of culture and the professional field, and it tends to reflect the values of the dominant society. Psychology students and professionals are taught to think psychologically (i.e., in accordance with the dominant psychological assumptions of the field) without critically thinking about the knowledge being deposited into one's mind. These psychologically educated professionals then rely on this acquired knowledge and impose a values system on clients that includes how they should see the good life and the outcomes they should want and seek from therapy.

EH psychology relies on a phenomenological method. Phenomenological methods provide an alternative to the dominant methods of the field, which can help shift toward a liberatory framework. Case formulation generally relies on interpretation. In most psychological frameworks, interpretation is made through theory and/or research. In other words, theory and research are the lens through which therapists understand their clients. Phenomenological methods, in contrast, attempt to understand the client apart from theory. That is, therapists using a phenomenological method seek to understand the client in the context of their experience. Phenomenology teaches one to bracket off their assumptions, including theory-based assumptions, to prevent these from tainting one's understanding. Research and knowledge still help the therapist recognize possibilities, but it should not determine the interpretation.

For example, in classical psychoanalytic theory, a therapist may assume, according to client disclosures, that a transference process is occurring. While a psychoanalytic therapist often tries to help the client uncover this on their own, the theory guides the psychoanalytic therapist's interactions in trying to uncover this. If the client does not recognize the transference process, the psychoanalyst may offer an interpretation with an assumption that the interpretation is, or almost surely is, correct because it is based on psychoanalytic theory. Conversely, in EH therapy, theory may help recognize a relational dynamic consistent with what psychoanalytic therapists and some EH therapists refer to as transference. However, EH therapists generally avoid assuming it is transference solely from reliance on the theory and instead focus on further exploring this dynamic with the client while maintaining an openness to other possibilities. To be fair, many psychoanalytic therapists, particularly contemporary psychoanalytic therapists, now also strive to remain open to other possibilities.

A second example is that in cognitive behavior theory, the therapist may assume that negative thoughts or thought patterns are the cause of the client's depression. The therapist may initiate interventions that inform the client that this is the reason for their depression—or a primary reason for it—and then initiate interventions to challenge these negative thoughts or thought patterns. An EH therapist may recognize thought patterns and highlight them, but they are less likely to assume that negative thoughts or thought patterns are the cause of the depression. Furthermore, they may not even assume the thought patterns are negative—what one person perceives as negative, another person may perceive as realistic or even see some optimism within the negative. Thus, the EH therapist is likely to be curious about the negative thought pattern and may explore it, but they will be cautious with their assumptions.

The examples articulated previously, like many examples, require some oversimplification, as is common with most examples. Yet, they illustrate the different uses of theory. A brief case example may further illustrate how theory can inform the therapist of possibilities without determining what is occurring. Hao recently moved to the United States from China for a job opportunity.[1] A recent graduate, he hoped to move back to China eventually. He began therapy due to distress resulting from adjusting to living in the United States. His therapist, Dr. Smith, was White and had lived in the United States his entire life. He was not familiar with Chinese culture, including the importance of filial piety[2] and family dynamics. Hao discussed the struggle of getting to work because he did not have a car and the bus was unreliable. He was making a good salary but did not want to get a loan and was sending money back to his family in China regularly. His work colleagues and friends were critical of him for not buying a car, leading to some distance and conflict in these relationships. This led to Hao feeling more alone and isolated. He strove to avoid conflict, particularly at work and with his supervisors, which was also an important cultural value. Not being familiar with Chinese culture or the concept of alienation, Dr. Smith did not recognize that the client was feeling alienated, which was a significant part of Hao's depression. Instead, Dr. Smith wondered if the client was struggling with dependency issues and explored this. After

---

[1] All case examples in this book are fictionalized and do not include details of real individuals to maintain confidentiality.
[2] Filial piety is a common value in China, derived largely from Confucianism. It emphasizes the importance of respecting one's parents, family, and ancestors. Generally, this includes considering and often prioritizing them in one's decisions.

discussing this in a session, he concluded that Hao was, indeed, suffering from dependency issues and developed a treatment approach seeking to address this and strengthen his independence. Dr. Smith lacked the theory and knowledge to really "see" Hao.

Hao began to feel more alienated, including in his therapy. While not trying to lead Hao, Dr. Smith kept directing attention toward possible dependency issues while not seeing that Hao was struggling with clashing cultural values playing out in his relationships. Fortunately, Dr. Smith was in a consultation group. One of the group members provided information on Chinese culture and the importance of filial piety and respecting authority, while another discussed alienation, including how it was different but could lead to isolation, loneliness, and questioning of oneself and one's values. Being receptive to this information, Dr. Smith was able to see dynamics that previously eluded him due to a lack of cultural knowledge and theory. In the next sessions, this recognition deepened Dr. Smith's empathy and made it more accurate. It also helped Dr. Smith recognize and better bracket some of his assumptions rooted in cultural blind spots. Hao started to feel less alienated in therapy, resulting in an improved therapeutic alliance, allowing therapy to become more effective.

Using the phenomenological approach and not using theory to interpret can never be done perfectly. It is unrealistic—even potentially harmful—to assume that one can fully set aside their assumptions and biases. Furthermore, without some prior knowledge, one often will not see or recognize aspects of someone else's experience. Dr. Smith was open to cultural differences and tried to rely on cultural humility, but without adequate cultural knowledge, he "didn't know what he didn't know." The lack of adequate theory or knowledge can limit the therapist's vision or close their eyes to aspects of what is occurring, which potentially can be just as harmful as overreliance on theory.

From an EH perspective, the therapist needs to hold on loosely to theory, allowing it to inform and help see possibilities in the client without determining how the client is seen or understood. There is a continual tension that the EH therapist must hold to accomplish this. It is not easy, especially when one resonates with or is excited about a theory. Thus, it is important to have knowledge about cultures and theories while concurrently having the skill to use this knowledge in a manner that informs without determining.

This discussion illustrates why it is imperative to recognize phenomenology as having a liberatory potential, not a given. In EH case formulation, the aim is to understand clients as they are without reliance on theory (paradoxically requiring some theory, knowledge, and skill), which enhances the liberatory potential. The phenomenological method, in itself, is insufficient to decolonize case formulation. There is a potential for bias that remains implicit. Frantz Fanon (1952/2008), who did the first phenomenological study of anti-Black racism in his book *Black Skin, White Masks*, critiqued aspects of phenomenology as insufficient without recognition of certain cultural dynamics embedded in a racist and colonized world. Fanon (1963/2004) maintained that "challenging the colonial world is not a rational confrontation of viewpoints. It is not a discourse on the universal, but the impassioned claim by the colonized that their world is fundamentally different" (p. 6). This demonstrates that any claim of universals risks alienation, colonization, and the imposition of values. Elsewhere, Fanon (1952/2008) stated, "A normal black child, having grown up with a normal family, will become abnormal at the slightest contact with the white world" (p. 122). This statement is essentially true, by definition, given that the cultural norms are different. However, Fanon considered this beyond mere differences in norms. Drawing from Fanon, any attempt at decolonizing case formulation must begin with the awareness of these different worlds, norms, and experiences and how they impact the individual client and culture more generally.

Living in "different worlds" with different norms, combined with the pervasive experience of anti-Black racism, results in a *historico-racial* schema[3] (Fanon, 1952/2008). In discussing this, Mahendran (2022) stated,

> The historico-racial schema is the sedimented personal experience of anti-Black racism that a Black person endures. These are not memories imprinted on the brain but sedimented experiences that pre-delineate the exterior horizons of what is possible and what to anticipate in an anti-Black world. (p. 144)

While Fanon focused on anti-Black racism, this could be applied to other marginalized groups as well. These sedimented experiences are not pathology but a normal reaction to a pathological or at-risk environment. As Jackson (2020) stated in reference to Black children, "Our children are not at-risk; they are at-potential in at-risk environments" (p. 39). The historico-racial schema can lead to the experience of alienation, which can occur in psychotherapy, particularly when the therapist is not aware of this dynamic (Hoffman & Islam, 2026).

Whaley (2011) addressed these dynamics in assessing paranoia symptom expression. After noting that Black researchers and scholars advocate that there can be a healthy mistrust or cultural paranoia among Black individuals, he stated, "Clinicians' ability to differentiate between cultural and clinical dimensions of paranoid symptoms in Black patients may be a key factor in preventing psychiatric misdiagnosis" (p. 388). It could be added that the ability to make this differentiation is also important for case formulation. Whaley maintains that reliance on the *Diagnostic and Statistical Manual of Mental Disorders* (American Psychiatric Association, 2022) criteria without the use of cultural knowledge often results in misdiagnosis due to cultural bias, leading him to advocate for a multistage process of assessing paranoia and cultural bias. Yet, even attunement to cultural knowledge is not always sufficient, further emphasizing the importance of an evolving, fluid approach.

While the topic of decolonizing case formulation deserves an article, if not a book, of its own, we hope these initial considerations demonstrate that an

---

[3]This term is sometimes translated from French as the "historical-racial schema."

EH approach has the potential to be applied consistent with principles of decolonization. We believe there needs to be continued scholarship focused on identifying ways that colonization and racism implicitly and systemically impact case formulation.

WHAT THIS BOOK IS NOT

Case Formulation in Existential–Humanistic Therapy does not address generalized guidelines for case formulation; however, some aspects are integrated into this approach. Other volumes, such as Tracy Eells's (2015) book *Psychotherapy Case Formulation*, provide an in-depth overview of generalized approaches. The aspects of generalized approaches integrated as sections in the EH approach generally are briefer, given the wealth of information available elsewhere. Some of these sections, such as diagnosis, are optional in the EH approach. We do not provide examples of these, given that most professionals receive extensive training on these aspects of case formulation. The lack of more in-depth consideration and inclusion of examples is not intended to devalue these aspects of therapy; rather, we have selected to avoid redundancy and unnecessarily adding length to this volume.

This book is not a comprehensive overview of EH theory and therapy. While we discuss aspects of EH therapy, it is recommended that you have some foundational familiarity with EH theory and therapy. Instead of providing a more complete overview, we point to scholarship that covers the theory and application in more detail. For the theory and treatment, specific recommendations are included in Appendix B for the relevant sections of the case formulation. For therapy applications, recommendations are discussed in Chapter 2, which focuses on identifying and mapping EH interventions; additional suggestions are also included in Appendix B. For a more general overview of the theory and application, we recommend the following resources:

- *Existential–Humanistic Therapy* (2nd ed.) by Kirk J. Schneider and Orah T. Krug (2017)

- "Introduction to Existential-Humanistic Psychology in a Cross-Cultural Context" by Louis Hoffman (2019c)

- "Existential–Humanistic and Existential–Integrative Theory" by Kirk J. Schneider and Louis Hoffman (2024)

- "Existential-Humanistic and Existential-Integrative Therapy: Philosophy and Theory" by Kirk J. Schneider (2019a)

- "Existential-Humanistic and Existential-Integrative Therapy: Method and Practice" by Orah T. Krug (2019)

- *Supervision Essentials for Existential–Humanistic Therapy* by Orah T. Krug and Kirk J. Schneider (2016)

This book also does not address the evidence base for EH therapy. For that information, please refer to its companion, *The Evidence-Based Foundations of Existential–Humanistic Therapy* (Hoffman & Lac, 2025).

OVERVIEW OF THIS BOOK'S CONTENTS

Case Formulation in Existential–Humanistic Therapy is designed to integrate an overview of EH case formulation with examples. In Chapter 1, we provide a broad overview of EH case formulation. Chapter 2 provides an overview of EH interventions, including interventions, stances, and techniques. Chapter 3 introduces Rasheeda, a fictionalized client followed through the next four chapters. Chapters 4 to 7 outline the first four major sections of EH case formulation—brief holistic client narrative, concern or problem identification, theoretical aspects of case formulation, and treatment planning. We return to Rasheeda in these chapters, using her case to illustrate each section. The final section of the case formulation template, additional information, is not described in its own chapter because it is simply an open, unstructured repository for additional details that do not fit anywhere else in the template. Chapter 8 reviews the support for treatment approaches, stances, and/or techniques section, which describes how the case formulation can form a basis for demonstrating EH therapists' practices are consistent with evidence-based practice. While this is a subsection of the treatment planning section of the case formulation, we have included it as a separate chapter because it is not traditionally included in a treatment plan. The companion volume to this book, *The Evidence-Based Foundations of Existential–Humanistic Therapy* (Hoffman & Lac, 2025), provides more detail about how EH therapy aligns with the three pillars of evidence-based practice in psychology: (a) the best available research; (b) clinical experience; and (c) client characteristics, culture, and preference. Chapter 9 provides several case illustrations of EH case formulations with different clients. The epilogue briefly summarizes the case formation approach covered by this book and its adaptability. Appendix A is the template developed for EH case formulation. Appendix B provides resources for individuals seeking to dig deeper into topics covered in the EH case formulation approach, such as the existential givens and the daimonic.

1

A Framework for Existential–Humanistic Case Formulation

Existential–humanistic (EH) case formulation draws on decades of theory, research, and clinical practice. The approach to EH case formulation we are proposing seeks to balance what is often required by insurance companies and many treatment settings with the uniqueness of an EH approach. We created a template that can be used to complete an EH case formulation (see Appendix A).[1] The template may be adapted in various ways, depending on the setting. In some settings, aspects of the case formulation may be excluded. For example, the *International Statistical Classification of Diseases and Related Health Problems* (*ICD-11*; World Health Organization, 2019) or *Diagnostic and Statistical Manual of Mental Disorders* (5th ed., text rev.; *DSM-5-TR*; American Psychiatric Association, 2022) diagnosis may be excluded in favor of diagnostic alternatives, such as the power threat meaning framework developed by Lucy Johnstone (2022; Johnstone & Boyle, 2018). In other settings, additional sections may be added, such as a "History of Substance Abuse" section in some treatment centers. In this chapter, we provide an overview of the approach to EH case formulation. We begin by discussing the stances and approaches important to EH case formulation. Next, we discuss the process and the sections included in EH case formulation. Finally, we discuss how this process evolves and is integrated into the therapy process.

---

[1]The template also can be downloaded from https://www.apa.org/pubs/books/case-formulation-existential-humanistic-therapy.

https://doi.org/10.1037/0000464-002
Case Formulation in Existential–Humanistic Therapy, by L. Hoffman and H. P. Cleare-Hoffman
Copyright © 2025 by the American Psychological Association. All rights reserved.

13

CASE FORMULATION STANCES AND APPROACHES

Several stances or approaches embedded in EH therapy are instrumental for case formulation. In this section, these stances are discussed, including presence, embodiment, phenomenological stance, and embodied curiosity. These strategies continue to be important throughout the therapy process. First, it is important to clarify what is meant by stances and approaches. EH therapy is often described as a techniqueless approach (Hoffman, 2019c). Arguably, this is overstated and dependent on how one defines techniques. In part, what EH therapy is trying to convey in stating that it is techniqueless is that it typically does not rely on structured or planned interventions carried out in specified ways at prescribed times. Of course, there are exceptions, such as in crisis situations. Instead, EH therapists strive to follow clients and be in tune with the moment-to-moment unfolding of the therapy process. At times, EH therapists guide clients or even direct clients to certain topics. For example, if the primary reason a client is entering therapy is grief that emerged from the death of a parent and this issue is not being discussed, the EH therapist may reflect that this topic has not been discussed in a session or for a couple of sessions to draw attention to this. Similarly, if a client is presenting for grief but other potential concerns, such as a relational conflict, appear evident, the therapist will explore these, potentially resulting in revising or expanding the focus of treatment if the client agrees. EH therapists also may integrate various techniques as appropriate. Most commonly, techniques more aligned with EH therapy are integrated, such as empty- or two-chair techniques, focusing techniques, or mindfulness techniques. As appropriate to the situation, EH therapists may integrate other techniques, even dialectical behavioral or other solution-focused techniques. When integrating techniques that do not align as closely with EH therapy, they generally are adapted to be used in a manner more consistent with EH therapy (see Hoffman, 2021). When more structured techniques are integrated into EH therapy, rarely are they planned. Rather, they emerge more organically or intuitively according to the flow of the session.

Instead of techniques, EH therapy is rooted in stances, conditions, approaches, or strategies that are more relational. Schneider and Krug (2017) stated, "These means, however, are not techniques in the classical sense; they are stances, or conditions, through which experiential liberation and profound transformation can take root" (p. 60). Many of these stances have significant overlap with the common factors of psychotherapy (see Wampold & Imel, 2015), which is why, in part, Wampold (2008) argued that EH therapy is as solidly rooted in the scientific evidence for psychotherapy effectiveness as any other approach. Similarly, what we refer to as strategies are more fluid than structured approaches. For example, phenomenological strategies, including bracketing, are used to facilitate exploration of the client's lived experience while limiting potential distortions from bias or theory. In this section, we do not consider all the EH stances or approaches used in therapy; rather, we focus on the stances and strategies most relevant to the case formulation process.

Presence

Schneider (2015) maintained that presence is the core factor in effective psychotherapy. Similarly, we advocate that presence forms an essential foundation for effective case formulation. Schneider (2015) defined presence as

> a complex mix of appreciative openness, concerted engagement, support, and expressiveness. . . . Presence performs both a holding, that is, containing function and an illuminating, that is, exploratory function; it both holds and illuminates that which is palpably significant within clients and between therapists and clients. (p. 305)

The holding and illuminating functions of presence are vital for helping clients and therapists collaboratively identify and clarify concerns that become the focus of EH therapy. We suggest absorption as an aspect of presence, which Wickramasekera (2007) described as entailing "extremely focused states of complete attentional involvement with their subjective experience" (p. 59). Wickramasekera found that the affective components of empathy are related to absorption.

Presence performs several roles in EH therapy, including being therapeutic in and of itself. Stated differently, the client's experience of the therapist's presence can be healing and facilitate growth. Presence also plays a vital role in establishing the therapeutic relationship, setting the context for therapy, and empowering other interventions. It is important, however, that it is not reduced to simply being something that one does to establish the relationship—it remains a vital part of EH therapy throughout the therapy process that directly contributes to change (see Krug et al., 2025). In case formulation, presence facilitates the process of inviting the client into a space of deeper reflection and engagement, thereby illuminating what is alive and palpable within themselves.

Embodiment Versus Technique

Carl Rogers (1980) developed one of the most important descriptions for becoming an effective humanistic (and existential–humanistic) therapist in discussing a way of being. For Rogers, therapy was about developing a way of being with others that is healing. This framework can be used to distinguish technique from embodied therapeutic strategies. By therapeutic technique, we mean a specific method or procedure that is intentionally employed similarly each time it is used to achieve a specified outcome or result. While techniques are adapted to the specific situation in which they are employed, they are implemented in a manner that is generally recognizable by an observer familiar with the specified technique. In many therapy approaches, techniques are either planned or employed when a particular issue emerges. Conversely, embodied therapeutic qualities are cultivated within the therapist to emerge naturally and fluidly within a relational context.

Elsewhere, I (Louis) illustrated this difference in reference to empathy (Hoffman, 2019c, 2020). In contemporary psychotherapy, empathy has often been reduced to a technique, such as empathetic statements or reflective listening. Students often have shared with us that they have been taught that empathy is something therapists do to build a good therapy relationship, with the implication being that empathy is something therapists do to build a relationship so that they can then do therapy. From an EH perspective, this is not empathy—at least, not embodied empathy. When empathy is embodied, it is something that the therapist feels or experiences from their experience of the client; it is a quality they have developed that emerges naturally in the therapeutic relationship. This embodied experience of empathy can be communicated to the client. The client's experience of empathy can be healing in and of itself. While empathy is not the whole of healing, it is consistently one aspect of the client's healing experience. This distinction between empathy as embodied versus being used as a technique has practical implications:

> When teaching about empathy I often ask students how they feel when someone uses empathy as a technique with them (Hoffman, 2019). Next, I ask how it feels when they experience someone being empathetic. I have used this questioning while teaching in four different countries and various contexts, yet the response is fairly consistent. When empathy has been used as a technique, the students typically identify responses of feeling dismissed and objectified, and their emotional reaction is often sadness, loneliness, and anger. When experiencing someone as being empathetic, they report feeling cared for and supported, and often describe this experience as healing. (Hoffman, 2020, p. 105; see also Kriz & Längle, 2012)

While the distinction between technique and embodiment is important for therapy, it is also relevant to case formulation. When case formulation is done to a client, it communicates something to the client and can lead to them feeling objectified. This often occurs when a therapist approaches the first sessions focused on obtaining history and details about the client and problem instead of getting to know them relationally. EH case formulation results from an engaged relationship with the client in which the therapist embodies curiosity, concern, and interest in the client. The information gathered to inform case formulation is sought relationally rather than through a structured interview. There are variations to this. At times, clients struggle to identify why they are coming to therapy or where to begin. Providing some structure early in the therapy process provides comfort that facilitates the process of getting to know the client. This may come in the form of inquiring or exploring aspects of the client's history.

Phenomenological Strategies or Stances

Phenomenological strategies or stances are foundational to an EH approach. At the outset, it is important to acknowledge that there are different approaches to phenomenology, and not all EH therapists or phenomenologists agree about all aspects of phenomenology, including how to apply it in therapy and research. However, a key aspect of phenomenology is trying to understand one's lived experience apart from prior theory. Much of psychology relies on interpreting clients' experiences through theory and research, while EH and phenomenological approaches try to understand the client's experience without reliance on prior theory. As discussed in the Introduction, this is one of the reasons EH therapists have long been averse to case formulation: Case formulation was seen as putting the therapist in the expert role and prioritizing theory and research over the client's subjective experience.

Phenomenology does not fit neatly with traditional approaches to case formulation. This was the biggest challenge we faced in developing an EH approach. However, it is possible to largely stay true to a phenomenological stance in case formulation. We say "largely" for several reasons. First, there are aspects of compromise between mainstream and EH approaches that shift the therapist from the phenomenological stance, such as when a *DSM* or *ICD* diagnosis is required or when treatment goals need to be consistent with the expectations or requirements of third-party payers or agencies. There also are times when it is appropriate to integrate more objective or expert stances, such as when assessing for suicidality and potential danger to others and addressing certain ethical or legal issues and when there are evident distortions of reality with the client. At times, it may even warrant integrating more objective measures. Similarly, it is important to integrate relational and other ways of knowing that may, at times, differ from phenomenology.

With therapy applications, EH therapists often go beyond phenomenological interventions, including the use of genuineness, the therapist's authenticity, and the real relationship in psychotherapy. Phenomenology is a primary EH stance but not the only one EH therapists use. This degree of reliance on phenomenology compared with other stances is one of the variations that exists between the existential therapies (see van Deurzen et al., 2019); there are also differences between different EH therapists regarding their degree of reliance on phenomenology.

Returning to the phenomenological method, it is important to unpack how this approach is used within EH therapy. When exploring the template (see Appendix A), there are many sections centered on EH theory, such as the existential givens. From an EH perspective, the existential givens are understood as universal challenges that all people encounter; however, these entail personal and cultural aspects regarding how they are experienced and responded to (Hoffman, 2019b). It still could be maintained that even identifying these as givens is, in essence, theory. However, EH therapists seek to minimize using the givens to interpret a client's experience and, instead, view these as aspects of life that everyone encounters. The therapist remains curious or open to how these givens may present themselves in the client's life.

The Role of Theory in Existential–Humanistic Psychotherapy

If theory is not used to interpret, what role does it play? From an EH perspective, theory helps us see instead of telling us what to see. A thought experiment may help to illustrate this. Imagine someone from 1000 AD being transported through time to 2025. Many things in the world today were never dreamed of 3,000 years ago. Never having seen a television, computer, or microwave before, the time traveler would be completely bewildered by these objects. Knowing what to do with them would be nearly impossible without some knowledge. As they talk with other people and learn about these objects, the objects become less mysterious, and the time traveler now better understands them. In this way, knowledge allows them to see what they could not otherwise see.

Another example may further illustrate this. Imagine a person who requires glasses to see. Without the glasses, everything—whether up close or at a distance—is blurry. With the glasses, the objects are clear. The glasses allow the person to see what is there (i.e., EH's use of theory to "see"). What is seen already existed in a blurred form, but they could not make sense of it without the aid of the glasses. This can be contrasted with smart glasses seen in some science fiction movies. Smart glasses help one see but also tell one what they are seeing (i.e., using theory to determine what one perceives). For example, when looking at a person, the glasses may bring up text or produce a voice in one's ear telling them who the person is and many details about their background. Both these examples are not without limitations, but they illustrate that theory is something to help one see. As the second illustration clarifies, theory helps one see without forcing a particular truth on what is seen.

An example closer to the topic at hand is the evolution of multicultural psychology, which provides a further illustration. Early approaches to teaching multicultural psychology focused on teaching about cultures and cultural differences by presenting information about different cultures (cf. banking model of education; Freire, 1970/2009). By imparting knowledge without critical thinking about what is being learned, knowledge often becomes more definitive and particular. When relying on knowledge about cultures to understand someone, biases and stereotypes emerge. Similarly, when one relies on theory to understand experience, assumptions follow that may distort the experience.

EH psychology has often been rooted in a different extreme, suggesting that EH therapists do not need to engage in multicultural issues because they focus on individuals' subjective experience—or their subjective experience, including their context (Hoffman et al., 2015). This is not sufficient. Without some cultural knowledge, therapists are not able to see some of the differences that exist. While rooting the idea of multicultural practice in knowledge of cultures is problematic, knowing how cultures can be different helps develop greater flexibility in one's understanding. For example, if a therapist has grown up in an individualist culture with no experience with people from collectivist cultures or education about collectivism, they will not be able to understand their client's experience or their own biases. To go further, if one has only had brief exposure to a single type of collectivism, one may miss the differences between different styles of collectivism that emerge within different cultures or even within a particular collectivist culture. While knowledge is not sufficient and must always be paired with other attitudes (i.e., cultural humility) and skill, some knowledge of differences has its place.

From an EH perspective, reading philosophy, theory, research, and different cultural perspectives is critical to expanding one's consciousness, awareness, and ability to see the variations in their clients' experiences. Two quotes from Rollo May are instructive here. First, he was fond of saying, "Read everything you can about psychology but leave it at the door when you enter the consulting room" (E. Mendelowitz, personal communication, October 19, 2017). Second, May often said that if you wanted to understand the cutting-edge understanding of what it means to be human, you should go to the literature department, not the psychology department (E. Mendelowitz, personal communication, October 19, 2017). May believed in reading broadly and not just psychology. This enriches individuals as people; however, it is important to be careful with how this knowledge is used. It provides a backdrop, but not a formula, for understanding and helping one's clients.

Embodied Curiosity

Curiosity is one of the most essential qualities of an EH therapist (Bugental, 1987). It is also a valuable quality for clients to cultivate that can be healing in itself while aiding in case formulation. Curiosity is not just a therapeutic technique but a therapeutic quality that therapists embody. If therapists are only curious enough to find the appropriate label or theoretical understanding of the problem (i.e., using curiosity as a technique) or use it primarily to convey interest to the client, they will miss important aspects of the client's experience and self-understanding while struggling to help clients cultivate this. Curiosity is most useful when embodied as part of one's way of being instead of as a therapeutic tool. When a therapist embodies curiosity, clients often become more curious about themselves and begin embodying curiosity as well. An important transition that frequently occurs in therapy is the client's shift from judgment or labeling of their own behavior or experience to being curious about them. An example may help illustrate this.

At the beginning of therapy, Juaquin frequently commented, "What is wrong with me? I am anxious all the time!"[2] He would follow this by asking for something to relieve the anxiety. As this kept emerging, each time his therapist would show curiosity about the anxiety, guiding Juaquin into his own curiosity. The anxiety decreased as the therapist engaged with curiosity, but the anxiety did not go away fully. After several sessions of this pattern, a shift occurred.

JUAQUIN: Last Friday, I noticed some anxiety when thinking about the coming weekend. I've been working nonstop for months and now finally had a weekend off. At first, I was frustrated, thinking that I should be excited for the weekend, not anxious. I started getting mad at myself for how I was feeling. I finally had time

---

[2]The case examples in this chapter are fictionalized and do not include details of real individuals to maintain confidentiality.

to slow down a minute, and I got anxious, ruining it. But then I realized my anxiety was because I had no plans. Yeah, I get to rest, but I will be resting by myself all weekend. I began wondering if this is why I work all the time—to keep me from being lonely and anxious.

THERAPIST: That seems important.

JUAQUIN: Yeah, but it's frustrating that I cannot tolerate a weekend by myself.

THERAPIST: I get that. It is not how you want to feel when you have time to yourself. At the same time, this helps clarify our focus here. You are starting to get a better sense of where your anxiety is coming from.

JUAQUIN: *[Eyes beginning to water, pausing.]* I was alone so much when I was growing up. Then, in college, I had this great friend group. But since moving here and taking this job, I'm alone again. At times, I feel like I did when I was growing up.

This brief illustration with Juaquin illuminates how the development of curiosity can have concurrent therapeutic and case formulation benefits. As Juaquin deepened his curiosity about himself, he began discovering what was underneath the anxiety. This created an emotional shift while clarifying the focus of treatment, which led to revisions in the initial case formulation.

Presence, the phenomenological stance, and embodied curiosity all require the therapist to stay open to being surprised and new possibilities emerging, helping to clarify the initial case formulation. Juaquin's anxiety did not resolve when he had the insight, but it did change. It became less intense while the sadness became more present.

THE PROCESS OF CASE FORMULATION

EH case formulation has been discussed as an ongoing process, and key aspects of EH therapy that inform the case formulation process have been considered. In this section, more specific skills for clarifying the concerns and problems and developing appropriate treatment strategies are considered.

Marking Patterns and Potential Concerns

Early sessions in psychotherapy are filled with possibilities. As a therapist, these possibilities can feel overwhelming; however, there is value in being patient and seeing what unfolds and clarifies instead of prematurely foreclosing on possibilities. *Marking* is used to help identify themes, patterns, and/or potential concerns to monitor them without forcing them into an interpretation or formulation. With marking, therapists identify potentially significant events to monitor, observing them to see if they emerge into something more specific and relevant. At other times, marking may identify a topic or potential theme to return to later. Saving these markers for later may be due to another issue being prominent, a client not being ready to go into a topic, or insufficient time to explore the topic fully (i.e., concerns that emerge at the end of a session). At times, the markers are vocalized (i.e., "That seems significant," "This theme seems to keep emerging"), or they may be a silent marker that the therapist notes to themselves to observe. Silent markers may refer to potential emergent themes or patterns when the therapist is not certain yet if they are significant.

Schneider and Krug (2017) discussed tagging and noting, which are similar to how we use markers and marking. For Schneider and Krug, noting is an aspect of vivifying resistance the first time that it occurs. Tagging is used to help identify repetitions of resistance. We are not differentiating between the first occurrence and subsequent occurrences nor restricting the use of markers to vivify resistance. However, noting and tagging could also be considered special types of marking. Stated differently, any notes or tags could also be considered markers.

Some markers may, over time, become clarified as not significant, while others are recognized as important. It is not necessary to know a marker is important to begin tracking it. Markers generally are exploratory, and the therapist is attending to them so that, together with the client, it can be determined if these warrant further consideration. If markers are determined with the client to be significant, both the therapist and client continue to highlight when this marker presents itself. The language of markers is generally not used with clients or even written out in case formulations; rather, they refer to the process of the therapist or the therapist and client recognizing something as potentially relevant and worthy of continued attention and consideration. Although the client is not using the language of markers or assisting with the case formulation, the therapist and client are often working together to identify themes that the therapist then identifies as markers.

Although it is not intended to be a comprehensive list, the following are several types of markers. It is not necessary or suggested to identify or label the type of marker when they are used. Rather, these are discussed to illustrate examples of what may be marked and how it may be used over time.

- *significant event markers*: This is marking an event that may be significant. For example, a client may discuss a breakup with a particular romantic partner in more detail or with more emotion than other prior romantic relationships. The therapist may mark this to continue attending to whether it is continuing to cause emotional distress or it is connected to other relational patterns.

- *emotion markers*: These refer to specific emotions or ways that emotions present or are described in therapy. Marking them helps the therapist or the therapist and client together attend to the frequency of the emotion and whether it may occur more frequently with particular topics or patterns.

- *nonverbal markers*: These refer to nonverbal forms of communication that occur. The client may or may not be aware of these. For example, clients may hold their breath or change their body posture. By marking these, the therapist may begin to recognize patterns when they emerge. The therapist may also reflect nonverbal behaviors to the client after they have presented themselves a few times so as to explore them together. These may connect with some of the following markers, such as pattern markers.

- *theme markers*: Particular themes, such as being devalued by oneself or others, may emerge. Marking them helps recognize if this theme often presents in proximity to certain topics, events, people, or other markers.

- *pattern markers*: These markers identify potential patterns the therapist is noticing. For example, if the client begins looking down and slowing down their rate of speech the first couple of times their sibling comes up, the therapist may mark this to continue noting or exploring.

- *therapy relationship markers*: These are occurrences in the therapy relationship that may be significant, such as potential idealization or devaluing of the therapist.

- *process markers*: These include markers related to process elements of therapy. For example, a marker can be used if a client changes topic each time the therapist reflects or comments on the client showing signs of anger.

- *here-and-now markers*: Like process and therapy relationship markers, these markers look for patterns and reactions to what is occurring in the here-and-now, either with the client or between the therapist and client.

Markers may be used in different ways. Here are some examples:

- *vocalized markers*: Vocalized markers are mentioned to the client. These can be more direct, such as saying, "This seems important. It may be good for us to dig deeper into this." Or they may be more subtle: "That seems significant."

- *silent markers*: Therapists may, at times, identify something potentially significant when it does not appear to be a good time to explore it. This may be due to the client not being ready, the lack of time, or the choice to follow a different theme that emerged in close proximity. The case formulation may note that these markers should be followed.

- *reflection of marker themes or patterns*: Here, the therapist reflects on how markers may fit together over time, which helps promote self-awareness. For example, the therapist may note, "Whenever you talk about Leon, you begin covering your face." Note that no interpretation is made with this reflection; it merely reflects the pattern.

- *interpretative markers*: As we have discussed, EH therapists tend to avoid interpreting through theory; however, there are times when they offer tentative interpretations through the client's experience to explore together. For example, a therapist working with a client struggling to understand their anger may say, "Your anger often emerges in situations where you feel unseen." While, depending on perspective, this may seem to be an interpretation, we refer to it here as an interpretative marker because it is something the therapist is continuing to explore, better understand, and confirm with the client. It is not something that the therapist assumes or determines to be true.

Connecting Markers

The use of markers is similar to coding in qualitative research. Saldaña (2016) stated, "A code in qualitative inquiry is most often a word or short phrase that symbolically assigns a summative, salient, essence-capturing, and/or evocative attribute for a portion of language-based or visual data . . . a researcher-generated construct that symbolizes or 'translates' data" (p. 4). There are different approaches to coding and grouping or coalescing codes to help identify units of meaning or patterns. Codes typically are used to generate primary and secondary themes that form the basis of the results in many approaches to qualitative research.

Similarly, in EH therapy, when something is identified as potentially relevant, it is marked (compared with an initial coding). If this does not emerge again, the therapist may recognize that it was not something significant and discontinue attending to it. However, the case formulation allows the therapist to step back and look at the markers to see if patterns emerge or if markers can be coalesced into potentially meaningful units. The markers may change or be relabeled, as often occurs in qualitative research as a theme becomes clearer. However, in EH therapy, they are rarely assumed to be accurate without confirmation from the client. Even then, the therapist and client remain open to new possibilities or interpretations.

How markers relate to other markers, such as their frequent co-occurrence, helps therapists and clients identify and clarify concerns or problems. Therapists across modalities, particularly depth psychology modalities, use processes similar to what we are describing with the use of markers. However, other approaches tend to connect markers with theory or structure-driven approaches. From an EH perspective, this is implemented in a client-centered manner, allowing the themes to emerge and be clarified through the client's and therapist's collaborative engagement with the process. The therapist should not be ahead of the client in the process but rather alongside them. In other words, although the therapist may be tracking themes and possible understandings, they do not come to conclusions about what is happening ahead of the client except in rare cases. Instead, as possibilities emerge, they are held loosely until confirmed with the client.

In seeking clarification or confirmation with the client, the therapist is not using the language of markers or presenting them as one might with qualitative research. Instead, the therapist does this in a more therapeutic language. The following are some examples of using markers in the service of clarification:

- "I notice when your father comes up here, you appear uncomfortable and look away. It seems he is difficult to talk about."

- "Often, when we start talking about the conflict with your partner, you smile and tell a joke. I am curious about that."

- "Have you noticed that whenever the topic of death comes up, it seems you begin to talk about your mother? I wonder if there is a connection."

Markers are also used to confirm a possibility that the therapist suggests. From an EH perspective, in many situations, it is preferential to use markers for clarification instead of confirmation because this is less likely to impose an interpretation on a client and more likely to embody curiosity. However, there may be times when a confirmation approach may be appropriate if the therapist phrases these gently and retains an openness to being surprised or corrected. The difference between these is subtle. The following are examples of using the markers for confirmation (these parallel the previous more exploratory examples):

- "When your father comes up, it appears to bring up feelings of guilt or shame in you."

- "It is difficult for you to talk about the conflict with your partner. When this comes up, you often deflect by telling a joke."

- "There seems to be a connection between your mother and death. Each time we discuss your death, your mother comes up."

When used for confirmation, statements are made as if they are likely true— a somewhat stronger statement than phrasing that leads explicitly with curiosity. Confirmation statements are still seeking further consideration or exploration. They are more effective when the client is comfortable correcting or disagreeing with the therapist.

Helping Clients Clarify Presenting Concerns and Focus

An important aspect of early therapy sessions is helping clients clarify their concerns and reasons for entering therapy. The client's initial presentation of their reasons for entering therapy is impacted by their understanding of what is appropriate for therapy. This understanding is often shaped by pop culture, including movies, television shows, and podcasts. Psychoanalytic or psycho-dynamic themes have significantly impacted how therapy is portrayed in pop culture and entertainment. Cognitive behavior therapy is frequently discussed in the news media, journals, and health magazines, which also then influences pop culture understanding. Therefore, clients often present with issues they feel are appropriate for therapy based on how therapy is represented in these media. Clients may also enter therapy due to a general sense of dis-ease or discomfort. They may recognize that something is not going well in their life but struggle to put this into words or make sense of it. At times, clients may not bring up issues or topics they believe are taboo or inappropriate for therapy. Or they may not discuss issues, fearing the therapist may judge either the client or a friend or family member who is contributing to their distress. Last, clients may not bring up their reasons for entering therapy initially because they have not developed sufficient trust in the therapist to feel safe discussing the real primary reason they are beginning treatment.

There are multiple reasons clients do not have clarity or feel safe disclosing their primary reasons for entering therapy. It is critical that therapists develop the ability to help clients clarify their reasons. Curiosity, the use of the phenomenological method, and presence are all valuable skills for clarifying presenting concerns; however, several other skills are particularly important to accomplishing this:

- being patient: Allow it to unfold and clarify at a pace that feels okay for the client.

- avoiding prematurely assuming clarity or understanding: When a possibility emerges, remain curious and open to other possibilities.

- facilitating continued exploration: In addition to remaining open to new possibilities, it is important that therapists help clients remain open to new issues or understanding their reasons for entering therapy.

- identifying patterns: This connects to marking, which was discussed earlier. Memory, or the appropriate use of notes[3] (including in the case formulation), is also an important aspect of this.

- finding language: Clients may not have the language to describe or clearly describe what they are struggling with. Therapists help clients find language that works for them. At times, this may align with common psychological, existential, or humanistic jargon. However, it is important to be cautious in imposing this language on clients. It is better to help clients find their own language, which may require therapists to develop a somewhat new language with each client.

Timelines, Fluidity, and Case Formulation as a Collaborative Aspect of Therapy

Eells (2015) noted that case formulation should be a fluid, ongoing process; however, in our experience, this rarely occurs, even when intended. Practices and policies at many clinics even subtly or not so subtly discourage this. It is

---

[3]This is not referring to taking notes in session, which is generally discouraged in EH therapy. Rather, it is talking about using case notes, process notes, or notes in the case formulation template.

also discouraged by the expectations of many insurance companies. The initial case report or case formulation is often supposed to be completed within five or eight sessions, sometimes after an initial psychodiagnostic intake session. The message in many training clinics and from insurance companies is that it is necessary to have a clear diagnosis, identification of the problem, and/or formulation after the first session and then implement a treatment approach from there. It is often suggested that it is a problem with the therapist if they cannot quickly diagnose and conceptualize the client's issues. Yet, as Yalom (2013) pointed out, it is often more difficult to diagnose after several sessions than after the first session. This is because, as the therapist gets to know a client better, more possibilities for what is causing the difficulties emerge.

The implication of the impetus to quickly diagnose and conceptualize is that the course of therapy should be set early, and rarely should the therapist diverge from it. Periodic updates are sometimes required after this; however, these rarely depart from the initial formulation, and when it does, this is often minor. This is partly because a diagnosis or formulation becomes a self-fulfilling prophecy (Yalom, 2013). In other words, a therapist interprets in accordance with the initial diagnosis or formulation instead of remaining open to new possibilities. Typically, updated reports focus on progress toward goals and changes in the client, potentially including new events impacting the client, but generally do so without rethinking the initial assumptions and plan developed in the first few sessions.

From an EH perspective, this process is problematic. Elkins (2009) noted that many clients do not reveal the primary reason they are entering therapy in the first session. They may feel unsafe revealing this before building a relationship with the therapist. Or, as one of my (Louis's) clients once posed, "You know those initial [intake] forms you have us complete? You know we lie on those?" While therapists may view this negatively, it is quite healthy. Therapists are not entitled to the trust of their clients based on their credentials and roles. To expect this from clients sends an unhealthy message that they should give trust to people before it is earned, particularly with people in authority. For some clients, trusting people who have not earned their trust is connected to the relational and emotional difficulties bringing them to therapy, including past traumas. Therapists feeling entitled to clients' trust can contribute to unhealthy dynamics in therapy, such as power differentials and pathologizing clients when they are not approaching therapy in the manner the therapist desires. Clients also may not be fully honest out of fear of insurance cutoffs or potential required disclosures to insurance companies. Elkins further suggested that, due to imposed limitations in the number of sessions or the therapist's own pressure to complete the course of treatment within a short number of sessions, therapists occasionally end therapy before the client reveals the primary issue or, at least, some of the issues prompting them to begin therapy.

The pressure to shorten the length of treatment or manualize treatment is not in the best interest of many clients or even third-party payers. Some research suggests that longer courses of therapy generally increase effectiveness for some, though not all, clients (Barkham & Lambert, 2021; Howard et al., 1986; Lambert & Archer, 2006; Shedler, 2010). Barkham and Lambert (2021) noted that "prespecified treatment lengths may not be a meaningful route to maximizing the effectiveness of psychological therapies" (p. 166). This is largely due to individual differences, which may also be useful in matching clients to appropriate therapy modalities and informing the pace of therapy. Thus, if a client ends therapy prematurely, it may result in continued psychological difficulties that may, in turn, impact their physical health. This prolongs the client's suffering, can contribute to hopelessness, and may increase health care costs through repeatedly returning to therapy and the psychological difficulties contributing to somatic or physical problems. Furthermore, clients may develop a belief that therapy is not designed to address certain issues and, instead, is designed for problems that can be addressed through brief and solution-focused approaches.

Manualized approaches also have limitations, including truncating any fluidity in the case formulation or therapy process. They generally require the case formulation to be established quickly and a manualized treatment map to be applied to the problem. Addis and Cardemil (2006) noted,

> Manuals provide an empirically incorrect map of the psychotherapy terrain that sends both research and practice in the wrong direction. The evidence does not support the assumption that specific therapist technical operations result in client change. Although training in manualized psychotherapies does enhance therapist learning of and technical competence in a given approach, no relationship exists between such manuals and outcome. (p. 148)

These manualized approaches do not reflect how therapy is generally practiced in the real world and are restricted in their ability to adapt to the specific client or emergent themes.

When early sessions are focused on information gathering, this sends a message to clients that can have a negative impact on them. First, this communicates that brief descriptions of the problem, diagnosis, and historical information are what are primarily useful. This impacts what the client presents in sessions. Second, this can be experienced as the therapist treating the client like an object or pathologizing the client. When the client becomes an object, the therapist becomes a technician addressing what is malfunctioning. Clients can experience this as alienating or even dehumanizing. Third, this works to establish a hierarchy with the therapist directing the process instead of establishing a more collaborative process.

From an EH perspective, the focus of the early sessions should be on establishing a good therapeutic alliance, trusting relationship, and collaborative process. There is a trust that what is important to emerge will naturally emerge, often over the course of the first eight to 12 sessions. Yet, sometimes, it may take several months for the client to feel safe enough to reveal their primary issues. The case formulation template may guide the therapist to recognize issues not emerging naturally through the process so that they can be intentionally addressed.

A brief example can help illustrate how recognizing missing information can be useful. Dr. Hugo had been seeing Stefan for 12 sessions. In reviewing the case formulation after the 12th session, he noticed that he had information about Stefan's wife, children, mother, and grandparents, but he had not mentioned his father beyond stating that his parents remained married. In the next session, Dr. Hugo commented, "I've noticed that most of your family has come up here, but we have not discussed your father much at all." Stefan looked away and became silent. When Dr. Hugo inquired, Stefan reported that they had a difficult relationship and that he had never brought this up with his previous therapists. His father worked a lot and was rarely home. When he made a playful comment about this in front of one of his friends, his father did not respond. However, as soon as his friend left, his father lectured him about being immature and not understanding why his father had to work so much. His father told Stefan never to speak negatively about him to anyone outside the family again. And he did not, not even with his previous therapists. After sharing this, Stefan reported feeling guilty for talking about this. Because a good therapeutic relationship had been established, Dr. Hugo's assurance that this would remain confidential and that it was important that he shared this calmed Stefan sufficiently, allowing him to begin exploring his relationship with his father more deeply in subsequent sessions.

Had Dr. Hugo asked about his father when gathering information at the beginning of the first session, Stefan likely would have glossed over his relationship with his father, and it is unlikely that the same depth of information would have been gathered. From what he shared, this is what happened in previous therapy experiences. By Session 13, Stefan trusted Dr. Hugo enough to go beyond what he had shared early on. Furthermore, the process leading up to the disclosures and his reaction in the moment provided important context that would have eluded Dr. Hugo had he focused on learning about Stefan's father through an information-gathering process at the beginning of therapy.

SECTIONS OF THE CASE FORMULATION TEMPLATE

The EH case formulation template (see Appendix A) is divided into five sections: (a) Brief Holistic Client Narrative, (b) Concern or Problem Identification, (c) Theoretical Aspects of the Case Formulation, (d) Treatment Planning, and (e) Additional Information. There are subtleties in this outline that have important implications. For example, the first section is separated from all other sections with no subsections and focuses on a holistic narrative of the client. From an EH perspective, it is crucial to see the person as a whole and not just focus on the problems. Often, case formulation focuses solely on the problem or development of the problem. Even the history gathered is generally centered on the problem. While it is important to understand the history of the presenting concern, therapists understand this differently if they look first at the problem. As noted by R. D. Laing (1969), "To look and to listen to a patient and to see 'signs' of schizophrenia as a 'disease' and to look and listen to him simply as a human being are to see and to hear in . . . radically different ways" (p. 33). This can be applied to any "disorder" in the *DSM-5-TR* or *ICD-11*. Therefore, we begin with a separate section on a holistic introduction to the client to frame how the client is seen and understood.

The second section is Concern or Problem Identification. The typical language in mainstream psychology approaches would just state the "problem." Adding "concern" broadens and potentially softens the possibilities of why a client is coming to therapy. For example, some clients may come to therapy primarily for personal growth and development, to deepen their understanding of themselves, as a preventive measure, or for other less clinical reasons. While third-party payers may be less likely to pay for therapy initiated for these reasons, they remain valid reasons for coming to therapy. Including concern also fits with EH's approach to avoid pathologizing the client. While some therapeutic orientations embed the problem within the case formulation, we have separated this. Again, the intent is to allow for a broader, more holistic understanding of the client in the formulation that is not solely centered around the problem. The Concern or Problem Identification section integrates some mainstream expectations with EH-specific perspectives.

The third section is Theoretical Aspects of Case Formulation. The early subsections are more generalist (i.e., client strengths, biological and physical considerations, family and social considerations, etc.), and later subsections are more EH specific (i.e., the here-and-now, the existential givens, etc.). A new wrinkle is integrated within each subsection: "Areas to Follow Up or Clarify." This distinguishes between possibilities or hypotheses and what has been confirmed or clarified with the client. These possibilities and hypotheses can include the markers discussed previously and possible ways these markers are related. Often, case formulation content begins in the section Areas to Follow Up or Clarify, then, after more exploration with the client, is moved to the main subsection. From an EH perspective, the client is generally understood as the expert on their experience, while most approaches to case formulation rely on the therapist as the expert on the client's experience. The Areas to Follow Up or Clarify distinction is crucial in creating a more fluid approach to case formulation that is consistent with EH therapy's foundation. Furthermore, this helps track markers and possibilities.

The fourth section is the Treatment Planning section. This again reflects an integration of what is expected in many treatment contexts and by third-party payers with EH-specific approaches. Therefore, a distinction is made between what clients may view as their desired goals or outcomes and the therapeutic goals and outcomes that are required to be sought in many settings and by third-party payers. This is seen in both the goals and intervention subsections. An important addition is the final section: Support for Treatment Approaches, Stances, and/or Techniques. Unfortunately, a common misperception in the field is that there is no empirical support for EH therapy (Hoffman, 2024, 2025; Hoffman et al., 2015). This final section is included to help EH therapists demonstrate that they are practicing consistent with evidence-based practice principles. A companion volume to this book is also being published to assist with this: *The Evidence-Based Foundations of Existential–Humanistic Therapy* (Hoffman & Lac, 2025).

The fifth and final section is simply "Additional Information." While this may seem obvious and unnecessary, it is important from an EH perspective because it helps root the approach in humility, including cultural and theoretical humility, and greater flexibility. Often, considerations may emerge with clients that do not neatly fit into the categories that mental health systems and professionals have created to understand clients better and guide treatment. This section is both a statement of recognition of these limitations and a space to explore and integrate perspectives beyond what is typically considered.

The template can be used in various ways. The primary approach we recommend is writing out the case formulation as a narrative, except for the Areas to Follow Up or Clarify section, which can be completed using bullet points. This is illustrated in the three examples in this book. This can easily be translated into a report by deleting the Areas to Follow Up or Clarify sections. In a report, many of the headings, particularly in the theory-specific sections, could be deleted to combine sections. If a report is not needed and this is being used solely as an aid to guide the therapy process, bullet points could be used on most or all sections. Using bullet points allows for quickly updating sections when information in the Areas to Follow Up or Clarify section has been clarified and/or confirmed with the client.

THE EVOLUTION OF CASE FORMULATION OVER THE COURSE OF TREATMENT

Although case formulation is an ongoing process, there are some changes in how it is engaged over time. In this section, we discuss ways that case formulation may evolve over the course of treatment. We divide this into (a) the first session, (b) early sessions, and (c) the ongoing process of case formulation. We do not include a specific number of sessions for these periods, nor do we suggest that they are stages of therapy. Rather, these represent fluid periods of therapy where the length of time spent on the relevant foci varies significantly from client to client.

The First Session

Consistent with emotion-focused therapy (Goldman & Greenberg, 2015), EH therapy "do[es] not separate the initial assessment phase from the initial therapy sessions" (p. 97). Beginning therapy and case formulation occur concurrently. The priorities in the first session include beginning to establish a good therapy relationship, engaging in therapy, assessing for the goodness of fit, and helping the client connect with hope or trust in the therapy process.

Establishing a Good Therapy Relationship and Engaging in Therapy
An important aspect of establishing a good therapeutic relationship is beginning to engage the therapy process from the start. Many core aspects of EH therapy, including presence, empathy, warmth, and genuineness, help establish a good therapy relationship. When therapy begins with an assessment process, it can feel objectifying and may communicate to the client messages about what is expected or important in therapy, even if unintentionally. Therefore, EH emphasizes the importance of beginning by engaging in the therapy process, which helps the client gain a more accurate sense of what therapy will be like.

Attending to certain factors in the first session and sometimes the first several sessions informs the early pace of therapy. For some clients, such as clients with prior bad experiences in therapy, a history of trauma, or difficulty with emotional regulation, a slower pace may be beneficial. Attending to the client's comfort with silence, exploring the here-and-now, and being with and expressing emotions, as well as considering their openness to revising or correcting the therapist's reflections or interpretations, informs the pace of therapy and case formulation. They also are important sources of information for clarifying client concerns or problems.

Assessing for the Goodness of Fit
The first session should assess for the goodness of fit from both the therapist's and the client's perspective. From an EH perspective, the goodness of fit is less concerned with the presenting issue and, instead, is focused on the client's values and desired outcome. Some of this may be evident quickly. For example, if the client is primarily seeking the development of skills, such as coping and problem-solving skills, it may be readily apparent that they are not a good fit for EH therapy and may benefit from a referral to a solution-focused therapist. However, at times, the focus on coping and skill development may represent the client's initial or urgent needs while the client also is interested in depth work. Wolfe (2008), for example, noted that for many clients with anxiety disorders, the first phase of therapy may be addressing the anxiety through a cognitive behavior approach before shifting to a focus on existential issues. Similarly, Hoffman (2021) advocated that when working with disaster response and trauma, it may be necessary to help the client develop adequate coping or emotional regulation skills to attain sufficient confidence in their ability to manage difficult emotions before focusing on the trauma. Therefore, in assessing for goodness of fit, it is important to look beyond the immediate needs or goals.

An essential part of assessing for the goodness of fit emerges through introducing the client to EH therapy. We recommend allowing at least 10 to 15 minutes to discuss this at the end of the first session. Often, this may begin by saying, for example, "In the first session, I like to share a bit about my approach to therapy to ensure that this feels like a good fit. Would it be okay if I did this now?" Clients typically agree to this; however, how much a client is able to take this in may vary. For example, some clients' first session is anxiety provoking, making it difficult to retain or process what the therapist shares. If this is the case, it is important for the therapist to note it. This provides information about the client that may be relevant to clarifying the problems, concerns, and patterns. In addition, if the client struggles to take in this information, it is valuable to revisit it over the next several sessions at a slower pace. Even if a client can manage the information, it is unlikely that they will remember all of it. Thus, it still will be important to revisit some important aspects. The following is an example of a brief introduction to the therapy approach:

> Although it is a bit of an oversimplification, the different approaches to therapy can be grouped into two general categories. The first is solution-focused therapy, which focuses on coping, skill development, and changing one's thoughts and behaviors. The second group could be called the depth psychotherapies. These approaches focus on helping develop a deeper understanding of yourself, your relationships, and how you want to live your life. From this deeper understanding, therapy seeks to help you make changes that address the deeper causes of the concerns or problems that brought you to therapy. I use the latter approach; however, there are times when I integrate aspects of solution-focused therapies as needed. As part of the depth approach, I believe the therapy relationship is the foundation for the work we will be doing together. Research suggests that the therapy relationship is an important part of the change and that if we can maintain a good therapy relationship, therapy will be beneficial more often than not.
>
> It is common to have thoughts and feelings about therapy or your therapist that may not initially make sense and sometimes may seem out of place. If this occurs, I encourage you to bring this up because it helps us to maintain a good therapy relationship. As part of this, I suggest two foundations for our work. If you ever wonder why I am doing something, please ask, and I will give you an honest answer. Second, if you ever wonder how I am reacting to something you say or how I feel about you or our therapy process, ask, and I will give an honest answer. At times, I may have to reflect a bit to give an honest answer to these questions.
>
> I generally do not give specific homework assignments often, such as worksheets to fill out. However, I will encourage you to spend time reflecting on or journaling about a topic. Occasionally, I may encourage you to write something to help you think through an issue or how you may want to communicate something to someone in your life. But there is always flexibility with how you approach this. I encourage you to pay attention to your dreams and write them down. While we do not always get a clear meaning from exploring dreams, even when we do not find a meaning, they can help identify concerns that need attention or are related to why you are coming to therapy. Do you have any questions about this or the therapy process in general?

After sharing about the approach and answering any questions the client may have relevant to this, we recommend asking the client if this feels like a good fit for what they are looking for. We are not recommending that you memorize or use the previous statement; rather, it is an example of how one may approach the first session. It should be adapted for the individual client. Some EH therapists may not feel comfortable with aspects of this, such as offering to share their reactions with the client or feelings about the client. If so, this can be omitted. However, before omitting it, therapists are encouraged to reflect on why they are omitting it to ensure it is not just discomfort or avoid-ance that would be better addressed through self-reflection. Therapists learning this approach may not feel comfortable including some of these statements, such as being willing to respond to questions about how the therapist feels toward the client. This may be something to aspire to once one is more expe-rienced. In addition, some EH therapists may want to add additional informa-tion; however, we recommend trying to keep this to no longer than 2 to 3 minutes to introduce the approach. The rest of the 10 to 15 minutes can be used for clarification or any questions the client has, along with a few of the following items.

If the client agrees this is a good fit, a few more issues are addressed. First, the client is provided with a rough estimate of the length of treatment. This may vary depending on the setting and presenting issues. In private practice, therapists may indicate that most clients come to therapy for between 6 months and 2 to 3 years, depending on the issues. However, the therapist may also clarify that when therapy is a longer process, there generally is significant improvement earlier in therapy. Even when clients are in therapy for a couple of years or longer, such as in the case of severe, prolonged, or complicated trauma, there typically is significant symptom reduction within the first 6 months of treatment.

Next, it is often important to discuss diagnosis, particularly if the client plans to use insurance. In some situations, this may not be necessary if a diagnosis is not needed. In such situations, the case formulation may replace the diagnosis (see Johnstone, 2018). If a diagnosis is needed or beneficial, it is important to discuss a possible preliminary diagnosis. As diagnosis is something that becomes part of a client's chart and can have an impact on a client, it is important to discuss the implications of receiving a diagnosis. In most situations, it is good to let the client know that, as the therapist gets to know them better, it may result in clarifications about the client that lead to a change in the diagnosis. The specific changes should be discussed with the client as well.

Connecting With Hope

Helping a client connect with hope is critical for the first session. The belief that therapy will be effective predicts better therapy outcomes (Wampold & Imel, 2015). Establishing this hope and belief that therapy will be beneficial in the first session or sessions bolsters therapy effectiveness and increases the likelihood that clients will continue in therapy. Often, establishing a good initial therapeutic alliance and providing an initial framework for therapy through the assessment of goodness of fit will be sufficient to instill hope. However, it is sometimes beneficial to provide additional sources of hope. This can be done in various ways. Frequently, it may be as simple as genuinely saying to the client, "I am confident that we can work together to address this issue and see improvement." If this is said in an embodied manner so that the client recognizes the confidence and hope in the therapist, it is particularly effective. Sometimes, it may be helpful to say, for example, "I have worked with people who have similar struggles before, and I am confident that we can address this together." Referencing past experience working with similar issues can bolster the client's confidence.

The Early Sessions

With the first session moving right into the therapy process, the early sessions build from this. The top priority is on establishing and deepening the therapy relationship. An important aspect of EH therapy includes what Mearns and Cooper (2017) referred to as working at relational depth, which they described stating,

> Relational depth in therapy can be characterised as a state of profound contact and engagement between therapist and client. Here, the therapist experiences high and consistent levels of both empathy and acceptance towards the client, and relates to them in a highly transparent way. Concomitantly, the client acknowledges the therapist's empathy, acceptance and congruence—either implicitly or explicitly—and is fully congruent in that moment. (p. 44)

While pacing with the client's comfort, moving toward relational depth is a priority. The EH therapist is consistently attending to the client's comfort moving into this depth by attending to nonverbals, observing the client's ability to work in the here-and-now (both intrapersonally and pertaining to the therapy relationship), being comfortable with silence, being open in self-disclosure, being able to disagree or correct the therapist, and being open to experience, staying with, and disclosing emotions. Moving toward relational depth is not only critical for therapy but also for case formulation. As greater relational depth is attained, it increases the client's willingness to explore and clarify concerns and problems. When relational depth is not attained, there is a greater likelihood that the client may not feel safe to disclose and explore reasons for entering therapy not recognized or disclosed in the first session.

In the early sessions, a priority for case formulation is remaining open to additional concerns and clarifying the concerns that have been shared. For example, if a client reported in the first session that they are entering therapy to decide whether to end their relationship with their partner, the early sessions may entail several dynamics. To begin with, the therapist may work to slow down the decision process, helping to ensure that the client can make a good, informed decision. The therapist seeks to attain a deeper understanding of the problem and how it is impacting the client in various domains, including interpersonally, emotionally, and at school or work. In addition, the therapist strives for a deeper sense of what the client has done to try to face or address the problem, as well as how they face problems in general. This often entails obtaining relevant information about how they handle relationship conflicts more generally and in previous romantic relationships. EH therapists also attend to how problematic relational patterns could emerge in the relationship with the therapist. This may include exploring with the client how they want to address difficult relational patterns if they emerge in the therapy relationship (i.e., preparing for or engaging with here-and-now work). The therapist also begins helping the client identify and clarify values relevant to this decision, including exploring how these values are relevant. While values clarification occasionally includes integrative strategies, such as using values inventories that are common in acceptance and commitment therapy (see Hayes et al., 2016), it is more common for EH therapists to strive to clarify values through the therapy relationship and engagement.

A foundation for the early sessions and the entire therapy process is remaining open to being surprised, potentially even expecting to be surprised. This radical openness helps therapists identify and explore issues that may be missed if they foreclose on their identification of the concerns or problems, assumptions pertaining to the etiology, or assumptions of factors causing the concern or problem. In terms of case formulation, the EH therapist begins taking notes on the case formulation template after the first session and continues adding notes, including various markers, until sufficient information is attained to write out the formal case formulation. Often, sufficient information is gathered within the first six to 12 sessions, but continual updating will remain necessary.

Occasionally, in the early sessions, it may become evident that aspects of history or context information are needed to clarify issues. This generally can be naturally addressed in the EH therapy process without needing to shift to a fact- or history-gathering approach. In the previous example with Stefan and Dr. Hugo, Dr. Hugo noted that Stefan's relationship with his father had not been discussed. By approaching this with curiosity, not a structured history gathering, the relational focus is retained.

The Ongoing Process of Case Formulation

We have emphasized that EH case formulation and treatment is an ongoing process. This should continue as an ongoing process through the final sessions, if not the final session. The ongoing process of case formulation relies on the same strategies discussed in the previous session, including remaining open to being surprised, embodying curiosity, continually updating one's formulation, and continuing to clarify and confirm possibilities with the client. Ideally, after the first eight to 12 sessions, the client will stay open to new possibilities and engage their problems with curiosity. As the therapist gets to know the client better and more concerns and possibilities are marked, the therapist and client will have a clearer vision of what is or may be occurring with the client.

Different milestones in therapy provide opportunities for reflection and clarification. It is important for the therapist to check in routinely about progress, the therapy relationship, and whether there are any issues not being addressed. For example, a therapist may develop a routine of checking in with the client about these issues at the beginning of each month. This may entail statements such as, "We've been working together for 3 months now. I am curious if there are any concerns or issues we are not addressing that need attention." The therapist may include the exploration in a query embedded in the therapy relationship: "We've been working together now for several months. I wanted to check in with you about how we are doing."

Periodically, it is important to review progress. For example, the therapist may state, "We've been working together for a while now. I am seeing some progress, but I am curious if you are noticing changes as well." This accomplishes several purposes. First, it helps assess if the client agrees about the progress. If the client does not recognize progress or the therapist is incorrect, this is also valuable to know. Clarifying agreement on progress helps the therapist recognize why changes they perceive may not be experienced as change for the client. Conversely, this may be valuable in helping clients recognize progress they may not have noticed. Because change is often gradual, sometimes clients do not recognize the change themselves. Using markers and including these in case formulation helps identify, track, and clarify change.

Checking in for progress is an opportunity to assess for the emergence of new issues. Sometimes, as a client makes progress and some concerns are addressed, it opens space to recognize other concerns or problems that may have been hidden or not recognized. For example, a client working on difficulty connecting with their romantic partner may, as this issue resolves, recognize unresolved grief from the ending of a previous relationship.

Beginning to talk about the end of therapy is an important time for case formulation. If the presenting concerns or problems have been adequately addressed, it may be assumed that the case formulation is done. However, the discussion of ending therapy often brings to the fore issues that have not been recognized. A common example is that the ending of therapy may prompt awareness of unresolved grief or prior painful endings of relationships. Similarly, it can also prompt fears about the return of the concerns or problems that provoked them to begin therapy or fears about being able to manage life without therapy. At times, it prompts clients to want to address concerns or problems they had been avoiding disclosing. Therefore, it is critical that therapists continue the case formulation process until the client has graduated from therapy.

ABBREVIATED CASE FORMULATION PROCESS

Thus far, we have focused on how to ideally approach EH case formulation. However, various factors may prevent this from happening. For example, many placement or employment settings require initial paperwork, including a treatment plan, to be completed after the first session or after a shorter number of sessions than preferred from an EH perspective. In addition, some placement or employment settings require a comprehensive history and diagnosis in the first session. In this section, we briefly discuss two adaptations: (a) required initial history gathering and assessment sessions and (b) a shortened timeline for case reports.

Required Initial History Gathering and Assessment Session

As we have discussed, an initial history gathering and assessment session is required in many placement and employment settings. Often, this is understandable, even if not ideal. We have raised the concern that this can negatively impact the therapeutic relationship, cause the client to feel objectified or alienated, and send problematic or contradictory messages about what therapy will be like, including what is expected from the client or important for the therapy process. While not negating the risk, discussing this openly with the client often helps:

> Our first session will be different from our sessions moving forward. This setting requires that I gather extensive information about your history and the nature of the presenting concerns in the first session. My preference in an ideal situation would be to start getting to know you through what you feel is important for me to know and building trust between us. I will do my best to try to integrate some of this into our first session, but I did want to prepare you for what to expect in the first couple of sessions as well.

When possible, it is beneficial to have a longer first session when required to gather a more extensive history and conduct a more thorough diagnostic assessment. This allows for time to integrate a relational process, at least for portions of the first session. However, some settings may not allow for this to occur either.

Shortened Timeline

A similar strategy can be employed when there is a shorter timeline for the report. For instance, it is common to require the case formulation to be completed after three, five, or eight sessions. In this case, we recommend beginning the first session as one typically would in an ideal EH approach. Frequently, much or all of what is needed for the initial case formulation will naturally emerge through the therapy process. However, if important details have not been gathered by the session before the report is due, the EH therapist may relay to the client that, in the next session, they need to gather some specific information for paperwork that is due. This prepares the client for what may be experienced as a shift in the therapy process and relationship.

USING COLLABORATIVE CASE FORMULATION TO GUIDE EXISTENTIAL-HUMANISTIC PSYCHOTHERAPY

Case formulations are intended to guide treatment; however, how they do varies with the approach to case formulation. EH therapy is not planned out in advance but rather requires the therapist to respond moment to moment to what is present in the session. Therefore, case formulation remains a fluid process. At the same time, the case formulation prevents the therapy process from going astray or on tangents that may not be beneficial or relevant. Our intention in developing an EH approach to case formulation is to provide a basic, fluid structure that helps students, trainees, and professionals learn this approach to therapy, particularly clarifying the process of understanding and conceptualizing the client's concerns and problems while thoughtfully considering what stances, strategies, or techniques may be most appropriate. This includes helping students and trainees recognize when integrative strategies are appropriate. Instead of using case formulation to schedule or plan interventions, case formulation helps EH therapists remain aware of the possibilities and potentials in each moment.

In the Theoretical Aspects of the Case Formulation section, the Areas to Follow Up or Clarify section is where many of the markers that have not yet been clarified are listed or explored. These are the possibilities that are not confirmed with the client and help therapists track issues. These also support the therapist's memory and vision (i.e., helping recognize patterns and connections). When using the EH case formulation template, therapists can review this before sessions, which serves several purposes:

- It refreshes the therapist's memory, making it easier to recognize patterns.

- It maintains markers to help the therapist identify patterns and themes.

- It maintains curiosities and identifies potential missing information. If a domain in the case formulation section has no content, the EH therapist may remain curious about this. This could mean that this is not a significant area of concern, that themes relevant to this section have not yet emerged, or that content relevant to this section is being avoided or defended against. The therapist does not, on their own, determine why, but they remain curious about the possibilities.

- It tracks what should be clarified and confirmed with the client. As clarification or confirmation occurs, these points may be shifted from the Areas to Follow Up or Clarify section to the main section above it.

- It identifies possible stances, strategies, or interventions that may be beneficial.

In supervision, the EH case formulation template can be regularly reviewed and updated. This provides a structure, albeit a fluid structure, from which students learn to recognize patterns and themes. However, it is important that supervision not focus too much on the template, lest this distracts from the relational process of supervision and the facilitation of developing a relational process with clients. Rather, the template supplements supervision. The supervisor also helps the supervisee learn to recognize patterns and themes from the markers identified.

CONCLUSION

For those familiar with mainstream approaches to case formulation, the EH approach may feel like a dramatic shift. On the surface, and even when perusing the EH case formulation template, it may appear similar to mainstream approaches while focusing on different content areas. However, when delving deeper into the process, the more dramatic shifts are evident. In particular, a deeper collaboration in which the therapist is no longer presented as the expert over the client's experience and the embracement of a phenomeno-logical approach represents a different paradigm for knowing and approaching therapy and understanding the client. It also reduces, though does not elimi-nate, the hierarchical approach implicit in therapy. At the same time, we sought to introduce compromises, which become more evident in Chapters 3 to 7 as we walk through the EH case formulation template. These compromises provide a foundation for how EH therapy can work in a mainstream context while maintaining theoretical integrity.

2

Existential–Humanistic Treatment Approaches

Identifying and Mapping Interventions

Existential–humanistic (EH) therapy has been discussed as a techniqueless approach to therapy (see Hoffman, 2019c). While this does not mean that EH therapy does not do anything, it complicates discussing how it works and what happens in an EH therapy session. Furthermore, it creates a barrier for some students and trainees attempting to learn this modality. Students learning EH therapy sometimes report that they do not feel like they are doing much, even when it is evident that significant changes are occurring with the clients. Often, when trying to correct this by doing more, they recognize this is not helping the therapy process, and frequently, the increased "action" interferes with it. The feeling of not doing much is partially because no specific techniques are used. Mark Yang (2020) described a similar experience in his book on EH supervision:

> Paradoxically, one of the most difficult things that supervisees need to let go of is their desire to help or fix their clients. This is not to be confused with being unmotivated or not caring about their clients. It has more to do with supervisees getting out of their own way and/or getting out of their clients' way on the path to healing. It is about being intentionally non-intentional and willfully without will, choosing deliberate non-action or effortless action, and acting without premeditation. In other words, it's about the Taoist concept of Wu Wei. Other ways of understanding Wu Wei is intention and act being simultaneous, not forcing, not imposing, not interfering. Wu Wei has been described as non-doing, but it is not doing nothing. (p. 94)

In part, the emphasis on not using techniques depends on one's definition and understanding of technique. As discussed in Chapter 1, EH prefers "stances"

---

https://doi.org/10.1037/0000464-003
Case Formulation in Existential–Humanistic Therapy, by L. Hoffman and H. P. Cleare-Hoffman

or "approaches." In our view, there needs to be clearer guides to what EH therapists do to aid in training and research. The risk associated with this is that any discussion of what EH therapists do can easily be reified into a technique, as has been done with various humanistic and EH strategies that have been integrated into mainstream approaches (e.g., Hoffman 2019c, 2020). In this chapter, we use the word *interventions* to refer to techniques, approaches, procedures, and stances that are intentionally implemented in EH therapy to facilitate change within the client. Often, these are intentionally used by embodying them. In this book, we do not review these interventions in great depth. Rather, we point to resources for those interested in learning more about how to apply these interventions (see Appendix B).

In this chapter, we begin by using two strategies to identify primary EH interventions that are then synthesized into a small number of primary interventions. The primary interventions, therefore, have variants in how they can be applied. Next, we briefly discuss each of these primary interventions, including, at times, considering some microskills or microinterventions that comprise ways these interventions can be implemented, often without feeling like an intervention or technique. While we discuss some microskills and micro-interventions, this is an area we recommend for further development. We consider some examples of when each primary EH intervention would be valuable for clients.

IDENTIFYING EXISTENTIAL–HUMANISTIC INTERVENTIONS

In this section, two strategies are used to identify EH interventions. First, we review research conducted with people who identify as EH therapists. Second, interventions are identified from several of the most influential books on EH therapy. After this, a synthesis of these approaches is introduced.

Research on Identifying Existential–Humanistic Interventions

To clarify what EH therapists do in therapy, when developing this approach to case formulation we conducted research asking EH therapists to identify up to 10 of their most frequently used interventions (Hoffman & Cleare-Hoffman, 2017a). Twenty-one interventions were identified by at least five different respondents:

- relational processing (17)
- experiential techniques (16)
- empathy (14)
- acceptance or unconditional positive regard (13)
- active or reflective listening (12)
- creativity or creative arts (11)
- searching for or promoting self-awareness (10)
- here-and-now focus or processing (10)

- confrontation (10)
- authenticity (8)
- presence (8)
- empowerment or encouragement (8)
- interpretative approaches (7)
- focusing (7)
- mindfulness (7)
- working with resistance (6)
- humor (6)
- dream-work (6)
- developing rapport or a therapeutic alliance (5)
- curiosity (5)
- psychoeducation (5)

In identifying interventions, we attempted to stay close to the language of the respondents. Several of these bear similarities; later in the chapter, these will be synthesized into primary EH interventions.

Identifying Interventions in Primary Existential–Humanistic Texts

To further clarify the EH interventions commonly used, we reviewed several influential and comprehensive sources identifying primary interventions, regardless of whether they are referred to as interventions, techniques, or stances or otherwise labeled. The selection of these sources was informed by research on key influences on EH therapy (Cleare-Hoffman & Hoffman, 2017). The sources included were:

- *Existential–Humanistic Therapy, Second Edition* (Schneider & Krug, 2017)[1]
- *Psychotherapy Isn't What You Think* (Bugental, 1999)
- *The Art of the Psychotherapist* (Bugental, 1987)[2]
- "Contributions of Existential Psychotherapy" (May, 1958)
- "Existential-Humanistic and Existential-Integrative Therapy: Method and Practice" (Krug, 2019)
- "Introduction to Existential-Humanistic Psychology in a Cross-Cultural Context" (Hoffman, 2019c)

In addition to these six overviews of EH therapy, we also included *Working at Relational Depth in Counseling and Psychotherapy* by Dave Mearns and Mick Cooper (2017). Although Mearns and Cooper are explicit that their approach is not tied to any particular theoretical orientation, we view working at relational depth as consistent with and essential to EH therapy.

---

[1]A third edition of *Existential–Humanistic Therapy* (Schneider & Krug, 2026) is being developed as this book goes to press.
[2]Bugental did not intend this as a book purely on EH psychotherapy; rather, he wrote it as a book on life-changing psychotherapies, which could include other depth-oriented approaches. We are intentionally selective about the interventions identified in this book.

While there are other overviews of EH therapy, many of these include the same scholars, and adding the additional sources would not add further interventions. With some of these approaches, particularly Schneider and Krug (2017), Hoffman (2019c), and Mearns and Cooper (2017), the language from the book or chapter was retained. With other overviews, including May (1958), Bugental (1987, 1999), and, to a degree, Krug (2019), a different language than what was presented in books or chapters was occasionally used. This was partly because the EH approach discussed in these books and chapters did not clearly label the interventions. A summary of the interventions identified are listed in Table 2.1.

The initial identification of interventions has significant overlap, at times with slightly different language. Therefore, we synthesized these interventions into a smaller set of primary interventions based on this identification of interventions. Some of the specific interventions were listed under multiple synthesized interventions due to the overlap of concepts. However, other conceptual overlaps were left separate. For example, presence could include empathy, genuineness, authenticity, and acceptance or positive regard; however, it is also more than this. The synthesized interventions are listed in Table 2.2 and are described in more detail later in this chapter.

The synthesized interventions intentionally line up well with the primary stances identified in the companion volume to this book, *The Evidence-Based Foundations of Existential–Humanistic Therapy* (Hoffman & Lac, 2025): therapeutic presence; empathy; working with emotions; authenticity, self-awareness, and facing life directly; here-and-now; meaning in life; acceptance; genuineness and the real relationship; self-disclosure; and the self. Others fall under "integrative strategies": mindfulness, creative and expressive arts, experiential techniques, and EH approaches to equine-facilitated psychotherapy. Two of these stances are not included in this chapter: the self and EH approaches to equine-facilitated psychotherapy. While the understanding of the self is not listed here in the interventions, it is related to many of these, including self-awareness. Existential–humanistic approaches to equine-facilitated psychotherapy similarly draw on many of the synthesized interventions identified (Vincent & Lac, 2025).

Some synthesized interventions were not included in the chapters in *The Evidence-Based Foundations of Existential–Humanistic Therapy* (Hoffman & Lac, 2025): understanding and working with protections or resistance and using objective or guiding stances or psychoeducation. These interventions were not included primarily due to difficulty identifying relevant research and overlap with other interventions.

PRIMARY EXISTENTIAL–HUMANISTIC INTERVENTIONS

Many EH interventions or stances sound deceptively simple, even basic; however, a more in-depth understanding of these recognizes that there is great complexity and nuance in learning to apply these intervention strategies effectively.

TABLE 2.1. Interventions Identified in Primary Existential–Humanistic Sources

Source	Interventions
Existential-Humanistic Therapy (Schneider & Krug, 2017)	• Presence • Identification of client's "battle" • Invoking the actual (attending to the side of the battle attempting to emerge) • Vivification of resistance and self-protections (attending to the side of the battle attempting to block emergent material) • Cultivation of counterwill • Coalescence of meaning, intentionality, and awe-embodied meditation • Noting and tagging • Embodied meditation
Psychotherapy Isn't What You Think (Bugental, 1999)	• Attending to experience • Clarifying meaning • Attending to the here-and-now or the present moment • Increasing self-knowledge and self-awareness • Searching • Working with resistance and self-protections • Shifting between objective and subjective stances
The Art of the Psychotherapist (Bugental, 1987)	• Presence • Interpersonal press • Paralleling (topical, feeling, frame, locus) • Shifting between objective and subjective stances • Working with resistance and self-protections • Moving in and out of emotion
"Contributions of Existential Psychotherapy" (May, 1958)	• Working with and listening to emotions (particularly anxiety and guilt) • Understanding the client in context (*Umwelt, Mitwelt, Eigenwelt*) • Promoting self-awareness • Presence • Facilitation of deepening the client's engagement with life
"Existential-Humanistic and Existential-Integrative Therapy: Method and Practice" (Krug, 2019)	• Sense-making and meaning-making • Working with protections and resistance • Facilitating awareness of the client's context • Presence

(continues)

TABLE 2.1. Interventions Identified in Primary Existential–Humanistic Sources (*Continued*)

Source	Interventions

"Introduction to Existential-Humanistic Psychology in a Cross-Cultural Context" (Hoffman, 2019c)	• Working with the client's existential context (i.e., existential givens)
	• Working with the daimonic
	• Presence
	• Empathy
	• Genuineness
	• Reflective listening
	• Working with emotions
	   – Processing (moving in and out of emotion)
	   – Listening to emotions
	• Experiential techniques
	• Normalizing
	• Facilitation of self-awareness
	• Facilitation of meaning
	• Creative arts interventions

Working at Relational Depth in Counseling and Psychotherapy (2nd ed.; Mearns & Cooper, 2017)	• Therapist awareness and capacity to interact • Positive regard and acceptance • Congruence • Empathy • Openness • Genuineness • Affirmation • Presence • Mutuality

TABLE 2.2. Synthesis of Existential–Humanistic Interventions

Synthesized primary EH interventions (stances, approaches, techniques, etc.)	EH interventions identified from primary texts
Presence	• Presence (Hoffman & Cleare-Hoffman, 2017a) • Presence (Schneider & Krug, 2017) • Presence (Bugental, 1987) • Presence (May, 1958) • Presence (Hoffman, 2019c) • Therapist awareness and capacity to interact (Mearns & Cooper, 2017) • Presence (Mearns & Cooper, 2017)
Empathy	• Empathy (Hoffman & Cleare-Hoffman, 2017a) • Empathy (Hoffman, 2019c) • Empathy (Mearns & Cooper, 2017)

TABLE 2.2. Synthesis of Existential–Humanistic Interventions (*Continued*)

Synthesized primary EH interventions (stances, approaches, techniques, etc.)	EH interventions identified from primary texts
Genuineness and the real relationship	• Empowerment and encouragement (Hoffman & Cleare-Hoffman, 2017a)
	• Humor (Hoffman & Cleare-Hoffman, 2017a)
	• Developing rapport or therapeutic alliance (Hoffman & Cleare-Hoffman, 2017a)
	• Genuineness (Hoffman, 2019c)
	• Congruence (Mearns & Cooper, 2017)
	• Affirmation (Mearns & Cooper, 2017)
	• Openness (Mearns & Cooper, 2017)
	• Mutuality (Mearns & Cooper, 2017)
Working with emotions, embodiment, and what is present	• Focusing (Hoffman & Cleare-Hoffman, 2017a)
	• Invoking the actual (Schneider & Krug, 2017)
	• Embodied meditation (Schneider & Krug, 2017)
	• Attending to emotions (Bugental, 1999)
	• Moving in and out of emotion (Bugental, 1987)
	• Working with and listening to emotions (particularly anxiety and guilt; May, 1958)
	• Working with the daimonic (Hoffman, 2019c)
	• Reflective listening (Hoffman, 2019c)
Authenticity, self-awareness, and facing life directly	• Searching for and promoting self-awareness (Hoffman & Cleare-Hoffman, 2017a)
	• Confrontation (Hoffman & Cleare-Hoffman, 2017a)
	• Authenticity (Hoffman & Cleare-Hoffman, 2017a)
	• Interpretative approaches (Hoffman & Cleare-Hoffman, 2017a)
	• Mindfulness (Hoffman & Cleare-Hoffman, 2017a)
	• Dreamwork (Hoffman & Cleare-Hoffman, 2017a)
	• Curiosity (Hoffman & Cleare-Hoffman, 2017a)
	• Embodied meditation (Schneider & Krug, 2017)
	• Noting and tagging (Schneider & Krug, 2017)
	• Increasing self-knowledge and self-awareness (Bugental, 1999)
	• Searching (Bugental, 1999)
	• Understanding the client in context (*Umwelt, Mitwelt, Eigenwelt*; May, 1958)
	• Promoting self-awareness (May, 1958)
	• Working with the client's existential context (i.e., existential givens; Hoffman, 2019c)
	• Working with the daimonic (Hoffman, 2019c)

(continues)

TABLE 2.2. Synthesis of Existential–Humanistic Interventions (*Continued*)

Synthesized primary EH interventions (stances, approaches, techniques, etc.)	EH interventions identified from primary texts

Understanding and working with protections and resistance	• Reflective listening (Hoffman, 2019c)
	• Working with emotions (Hoffman, 2019c)
	  – Processing (moving in and out of emotion)
	  – Listening to emotions
	• Facilitation of self-awareness (Hoffman, 2019c)
	• Confrontation (Hoffman & Cleare-Hoffman, 2017a)
	• Working with resistance (Hoffman & Cleare-Hoffman, 2017a)
	• Vivification of resistance and self-protections (Schneider & Krug, 2017)
	• Cultivation of counterwill (Schneider & Krug, 2017)
	• Identification of clients' "battle" (Schneider & Krug, 2017)
	• Noting and tagging (Schneider & Krug, 2017)
	• Working with resistance (Bugental 1987, 1999)

Meaning-centered interventions	• Coalescence of meaning, intentionality, and awe-embodied meditation (Schneider & Krug, 2017) • Clarifying meaning (Bugental, 1999) • Facilitation of meaning (Hoffman, 2019c)
Here-and-now	• Here-and-now processing (Hoffman & Cleare-Hoffman, 2017a) • Active and reflective listening (Hoffman & Cleare-Hoffman, 2017a) • Relational processing (Hoffman & Cleare-Hoffman, 2017a) • Attending to the here-and-now or present moment (Bugental, 1999) • Reflective listening (Hoffman, 2019c)
Self-disclosure	• Congruence (Mearns & Cooper, 2017) • Openness (Mearns & Cooper, 2017) • Mutuality (Mearns & Cooper, 2017)
Positive regard and acceptance	• Acceptance and unconditional positive regard (Hoffman & Cleare-Hoffman, 2017a) • Empowerment and encouragement (Hoffman & Cleare-Hoffman, 2017a) • Positive regard and acceptance (Mearns & Cooper, 2017) • Affirmation (Mearns & Cooper, 2017)
Utilizing objective or guiding stances and psychoeducation	• Psychoeducation (Hoffman & Cleare-Hoffman, 2017a) • Shifting between subjective and objective stances (Bugental, 1999) • Interpersonal press (Bugental, 1987)

TABLE 2.2. Synthesis of Existential-Humanistic Interventions (*Continued*)

Synthesized primary EH interventions (stances, approaches, techniques, etc.)	EH interventions identified from primary texts
Experiential techniques	• Experiential techniques (Hoffman & Cleare-Hoffman, 2017a)
	• Experiential techniques (Hoffman, 2019c)
Creative and expressive arts interventions	• Creativity and creative arts (Hoffman & Cleare-Hoffman, 2017a)
	• Creative arts interventions (Hoffman, 2019c)
Mindfulness	• Mindfulness (Hoffman & Cleare-Hoffman, 2017a)

Note. Several of these EH interventions could potentially fit in several synthesized primary EH intervention categories. EH = existential-humanistic.

Furthermore, the intent is generally to embody or integrate them into one's way of being with clients, not reduce them to simplified techniques. In this section, we provide a brief three- to four-paragraph introduction to each of the primary interventions and briefer overviews of the integrative interventions. Most of the primary interventions are discussed in more depth with consideration of supporting research and multicultural adaptations in *The Evidence-Based Foundations of Existential–Humanistic Therapy.*

Presence

The concept of presence can be traced back at least to Rollo May's (1958) chapter on the contributions of existential therapy in the book *Existence*, which introduced many in the United States to existential psychology. It has remained a foundational aspect of EH therapy since this time. Schneider and Krug (2017) defined presence as

> the capacity to be before or to be with one's being and to be before or to be with another human being. Presence assumes both availability and expressiveness. It holds and illuminates that which is palpably (immediately, affectively, kinesthetically, and profoundly) relevant within the client and between client and therapist. (pp. 192–193)

Presence could be understood as including or being closely related to empathy, genuineness, authenticity, acceptance, and other interventions; however, it is also more than these or the sum of these parts. In addition, qualities such as absorption are related to presence (see Wickramasekera, 2007). Presence is sometimes misunderstood as being "being fully present." While this can be a component of presence, presence is much more than just being fully present. For example, presence also includes expressiveness, genuineness, acceptance, and authenticity.

Schneider (2015) maintained that presence is the core contextual factor of therapy and the foundation for effective practice. As such, this is central to EH therapy across varied clients. However, as with all therapy stances and interventions, modification may be necessary for clients based on individual and cultural differences. As noted in the definition by Schneider and Krug (2017), an aspect of presence is a mutuality of being present with oneself and the other person. Therefore, it draws both therapist and client into being more present with themselves and the other person in the therapy dyad. For some clients, this feels overwhelming or even unsafe, especially at first. For example, a Black gay client who has experienced frequent racism and homophobia may feel uncomfortable with and resistant to presence with a White, heterosexual, cisgender therapist. While this may fade over time, it can be important for the therapist to begin with more objective and/or distanced stances and gradually work toward integrating presence when and if the client is more receptive to this.

Presence serves several purposes with clients. It helps clients recognize that they are not alone and are valued. However, presence also invites clients to open up to and deepen their awareness of their experience. This facilitates a deeper connection with themselves, including helping clients overcome self-alienation or intrapersonal isolation. As Schneider (2015) noted, it also illuminates the client's experience. Furthermore, presence can empower other interventions, including integrative interventions, such as solution-focused interventions, and other EH interventions, such as meaning-oriented strategies or interventions.

Empathy

Bohart and Greenberg (1997a) identified three primary categories of how empathy is understood: (a) empathetic rapport, (b) experience-near understanding of the client, and (c) communicative attunement. However, Hoffman (2020) noted that in mainstream approaches, empathy may be reduced to empathetic statements and understood merely as something therapists do to build trust and a therapeutic alliance. Conversely, for EH therapy, "Empathy also is healing in and of itself" (Hoffman, 2020, p. 104). Rogers (1959) described empathy as a state, which points toward empathy as part of the therapist's way of being with clients. Similarly, Mearns and Cooper (2017) discussed *embodied empathy*, which may include all three aspects of empathy identified by Bohart and Greenberg (1997a).

While empathy is, to a degree, experiencing what a client is experiencing, it is important that therapists do not lose their rootedness or groundedness in themselves because this would, according to Rogers (1959), signify a different experience than empathy. Also, as Hoffman (2020) emphasized, it is important that therapists do not assume that empathy is accurate, especially when working with clients from different social positions.

Therapists convey empathy in various ways, including voicing and showing the emotions the client is experiencing. Voicing is giving name to what the client is experiencing; however, this often is more effective if the therapist genuinely demonstrates that they are participating in the emotion with the client in some manner. When a client is crying, therapists may use a softened voice or show that they are impacted through facial expressions or eyes watering with tears. Similarly, when a client is angry, empathy may be conveyed by the therapist allowing themself to feel the anger as well, demonstrating this in a slightly raised voice or clenched jaw. As the empathy is conveyed, however, the therapist does not lose their ground, demonstrating to clients that one can be with the emotion without being overwhelmed by it. Therefore, the therapist can model how to contain emotions.

A therapist experiencing embodied empathy can be a powerful experience and serves several purposes, including, but not limited to, validating a client's experience, helping them deepen their exploration of their experience, and giving permission to feel emotions that a client has been resisting. It is valuable for clients who are struggling to accept and understand their emotions; experiencing isolation, loneliness, and/or alienation; and dissociating or repressing aspects of their experience.

Genuineness and the Real Relationship

Genuineness is a complex concept with some variations in how it is understood. From an EH perspective, Morrill (2025) described genuineness as a multifaceted construct "comprised of the therapist's self-awareness, presence, willingness to self-disclose, and emotional involvement in the client's story and the here-and-now interaction" (p. 269). In distinguishing it from authenticity, it is essentially interpersonal. The real relationship in psychotherapy is a closely related, though distinct, construct. Gelso and Silberberg (2016) described the real relationship as

> The personal or person-to-person relationship that exists between the psychotherapy participants from the moment of first contact, consisting of the extent to which they perceive/experience each other in a way that befits who they are (termed realism) and respond to each other in an authentic, nonphony manner (termed genuineness). (p. 154)

While some approaches, such as earlier models of psychoanalysis, view the relationship as largely comprising transferences, countertransferences, projections, and distortions, in EH therapy, while limitations are always present in relationships, there is a real relationship that exists between the therapist and client. Furthermore, this real relationship is valuable.

Like presence, genuineness and the real relationship in psychotherapy provide a foundation for the therapy relationship and other interventions while also serving as a powerful source of change. For instance, it is common for clients to dismiss—either internally or in direct statements—the therapist's concern, acceptance, or care as merely part of their professional role. When the therapy relationship is viewed as artificial or disingenuous, it limits and disempowers it. Helping the client experience the relationship as real or genuine provides a corrective relational experience that helps clients change how they experience other relationships (Stark, 2000).

Genuineness and the real relationship are important for clients who are struggling interpersonally due to past trauma, difficulties with trust, and other relational challenges. These are also important for clients who struggle with trusting themselves. In addition, genuineness and the real relationship help clients face difficult emotions and issues, knowing they are not alone. For example, in a demonstration that I (Louis) did many years ago, the person in the client role noted, "I could feel you urging me to go deeper, which was scary, but I could do it because I could tell you were right there with me."

Working With Emotions, Embodiment, and What Is Present

Emotions are part of being human. While many therapies primarily try to help clients manage or control emotions, EH therapy seeks to shift how clients experience emotions. At times, it is important for clients to develop coping or emotion regulation skills to be able to go into emotions and change their relationship with their emotions; however, the longer term intention is to help clients change their experience of emotions. A foundation, then, is the assertion that emotions, at their base, are healthy. While emotions can develop into problematic patterns, this does not mean that, at their core, they are pathological. When emotions are repressed or overcontrolled, they do not go away. Instead, the resistance to experiencing, processing, and listening to one's emotions often leads them to become more problematic.

EH approaches to working with emotions can take various trajectories (Varisco & Hoffman, 2025). Effectively working with emotions in EH therapy involves several factors, including pacing, timing, awareness of the client's current context, and determining if the client has sufficient resources for managing emotions. A primary aspect of EH approaches to working with emotions is emotional processing. Emotional processing includes awareness and experiencing one's emotions and reflecting on them, sense making, and meaning making. As part of this, clients will be moving in and out of their emotions (see Bugental, 1987), which in itself can facilitate emotional change. The EH therapist often uses different strategies to guide clients to go more deeply into their emotions and then step back to reflect on them, including sense-making and meaning-making. Curiosity—the therapist's and the cultivation of the client's curiosity—is an important therapeutic tool. Moving from resisting one's emotions to becoming curious about them serves several purposes. First, this shift often decreases the distress of emotions. Second, it helps clients understand their emotions and listen to messages or wisdom that may be inherent in their emotional responses. Rollo May (1950/1970, 1958) endorsed anxiety as an important guide for therapy. Recognizing anxiety as a guide can help clients experience what Schneider (2023) called *life-enhancing anxiety*. This can be applied to other emotions as well. As clients become curious about their emotions, the emotions guide therapy and can be experienced as life-enhancing.

Working with emotions is vital for many issues that emerge in therapy, including presenting issues that involve emotional distress or dysregulation.

While, as noted, the first part of helping clients address distressing emotions may be improving emotional regulation skills, this is not the end of therapy as it might be in some modalities. Rather, this is the inception of a new journey with one's emotions.

Authenticity, Self-Awareness, and Facing Life Directly

There are different understandings of authenticity in existential philosophy and psychology (see DuBose, 2026; Spaeth et al., 2025). In this book, we rely on the understanding of authenticity represented by Sartre and, in particular, Beauvoir (see Cleary, 2022; Spaeth et al., 2025). Unpacking authenticity clarifies how it relates to self-awareness and facing life directly. Ellenberger (1958) stated, "Authentic existence is the modality in which a man assumes the responsibility of his own existence" (p. 118). This is a foundation because it demonstrates that responsibility is essential for the existential condition of authenticity. For Bugental (1965), essential to taking responsibility is an awareness of one's existential condition, including facing the givens of existence, which connect authenticity with self-awareness and facing life directly. Cleary (2022), drawing from Beauvoir, pulls these together, stating,

> To become authentic means to create our own essence. It's the creation that is vital here. We don't discover ourselves, we make ourselves. Authenticity is a way of expressing our freedom: to realize and accept that we are free; to be lucid about what we can and can't choose about ourselves, our situation, and others; and to use our freedom as a tool to shape ourselves. (p. x)

For Beauvoir (1948/1976), authenticity also necessitates recognition of interconnectedness, including that one's freedom (and therefore responsibility) is connected to the freedom of others. This demonstrates that authenticity is a rich, complex topic in existential psychology.

This understanding of authenticity leads to the problem of ethical living, which, for Frankl (1946/1984, 2001), was closely connected to happiness. Frankl believed that happiness should not be pursued but viewed as an outcome of a well-lived, ethical life. While Frankl was not an EH therapist, this fits with an EH perspective. Therefore, one cannot pursue authenticity without consideration of the ethical dimension of life. But how does this connect with therapy interventions? From an EH perspective, the therapist's authenticity is a foundation for how they are in the world, including when they are with clients. This includes the therapist doing their own work (i.e., self-awareness, facing life directly) and honoring the client's freedom and responsibility. If therapists infringe on clients' freedom and responsibility by imposing decisions or values on them through therapy interventions, they are acting inauthentically. Thus, the EH therapist strives to cultivate freedom or choice within the client alongside them to promote taking responsibility for their lives. However, as Rollo May (1981) articulated, freedom must be understood in the context of destiny or the aspects of life that influence one beyond their control. Authenticity, then, also recognizes acting in the context of the limitations of one's freedom.

Xuefu Wang (2019) views facing life directly (i.e., zhi main) as including facing oneself, others, and the world directly. This is a complex understanding that includes various types of self-awareness as central to authentic living. While an aspect of facing life directly is a confrontation with the existential givens, caution is warranted. As noted by Vos (2025a), there are dangers in thrusting clients into the face of the givens. While facing the givens is not always significantly distressing, it can be. Therefore, several considerations are crucial. First, EH therapists do not lead or push clients to confront the givens; rather, when a client inevitably is drawn into facing one of the givens, the therapist sensitively assists the client with this confrontation. Second, EH therapists strive to assess if the client is ready to face the givens, including sufficient coping and supportive resources if needed. The strength of the therapeutic relationship is also an important consideration in readiness. At times, the therapist slows down the process until the client is ready.

EH therapists use various strategies, including phenomenological, searching, focusing, and mindfulness, to promote self-reflection and self-awareness. EH therapists also help clients recognize choices they are making without recognizing they are making a choice, as well as helping them make informed choices. An aspect of this, too, is clarifying the client's values and, as Schneider (2023) noted, how they are "willing to live" (p. 43). The development of authenticity overlaps with meaning-oriented interventions. This is particularly valuable for clients struggling with depression, trauma that includes an existential shattering, or life transitions. *Existential shattering* is a concept developed by Tom Greening that refers to the shattering of one's worldview or sense of security in the world (Hoffman & Vallejos, 2018). This is often sudden but can also be part of a gradual process building up to the shattering.

Understanding and Working With Protections and Resistance

Protections, in EH psychology, is an alternative term to resistance that seeks to depathologize what is often referred to as resistance (Bugental, 1999; Schneider & Krug, 2017). These are also similar to what psychoanalytic theory calls defense mechanisms. Protections are blocks emerging within the client or between the client and therapist. Often, these represent processes that the client has used to protect themselves. They may have served the client well at times and may continue to serve a beneficial purpose for the client at times. For example, a client may have learned to use humor as a protection in uncomfortable situations. This helped the client survive or manage difficult situations; however, now, they may occasionally use it when it is not needed or beneficial. From an EH perspective, everyone needs some protections. Therefore, instead of viewing these negatively or as harmful, protections should be recognized as having both the potential for benefit and harm. Various EH strategies can be incorporated when working with resistance.

Schneider and Krug (2017) discussed several strategies for working with resistance, including noting and tagging, which is part of vivifying resistance.

They define the vivification of resistance as the "intensification (or mirroring) of clients' awareness of how they block or limit themselves; vivification alerts clients to these blocks or limits, whereas confrontation alarms clients" (p. 194). To accomplish this, the therapist notes (the initial highlighting or mirroring of the protection) and tags (alerting or reflecting to the client ongoing patterns of protections) when protections are used. This heightened awareness empowers choice. Vivification of resistance also helps clients become more intentional about using protections (Hoffman, 2021; Jackson & Pintauro, 2026). For instance, drawing from the earlier example of humor, EH therapists may work to help the client use humor as a protection more intentionally, which can lead to using it more sparingly. This empowers clients to use natural coping mechanisms in a more productive and intentional manner.

Working with protections and resistance is closely related to authenticity, self-awareness, and facing life directly and could be considered a part of this. The issue of protection comes up rather pervasively with clients; therefore, it is relevant to nearly all clients who enter therapy. However, it may be particularly relevant for clients with strong patterns of avoidance or denial.

Meaning-Centered Interventions

Meaning has become one of the most studied concepts in psychology and therapy, with strong evidence supporting its role in promoting mental health (Vos, 2018, 2025b, 2026). Viktor Frankl (1946/1984, 2001), developer of logotherapy, is the existential therapist who most ardently advocated for the centrality of meaning. While EH therapists consider meaning alongside many other themes instead of as the central aspect of existential therapy, it remains important. For existential therapists, meaning refers to purpose or value, not sense-making, though sense-making may also be important in the pursuit of meaning. In addition, for EH therapists, the emphasis is on meaning in life, not the meaning of life. In other words, there is no central meaning that everyone must pursue; rather, various types of meaning can be pursued (Vos, 2018, 2025a, 2025b). Vos, a leading researcher on meaning, identified various types of meaning, some of which are more likely to be sustaining meanings or meanings that constructively contribute to the quality of life. These include materialistic types of meaning, hedonistic types, self-oriented types, social types, larger types, and existential-philosophical types. There are an additional 29 subtypes connected with these primary types. Vos and Vitali (2018) found that exploring more types and subtypes of meaning was associated with better therapy outcomes. In addition, Vos (2025a) found that the types of meaning typically sought and most effective may evolve over an individual's lifespan.

Schneider (2004, 2009, 2019b) advocated for the centrality of awe, which he connected with meaning. *Awe* can be defined as

> humility and wonder before the bigger picture of living, often attained by clients following the removal of blocks to their innermost sensibilities about life and their maximal ranges of experience. The sense of awe is an increasingly recognized

spiritual dimension of intensive existential–humanistic practice and a vital context for the optimal appreciation of life. (Schneider & Krug, 2017, p. 188)

The connection with or experience of awe can be a primary source of meaning in life. Although it is a less concrete form of meaning, it does not devalue awe or make it lesser than other forms of meaning. In therapy, an appreciation of awe can be cultivated with clients by helping them recognize and be with its presence or encouraging them to seek out sources of awe. Schneider and Krug (2017) stated, "By the cultivation of awe, we mean clients' renewed abilities to experience the fullness of their lives—their deepest dreads as well as their most dazzling desires—and their rejuvenated capacity for choice" (p. 100).

Vos (2018) identified various meaning-centered interventions that can be integrated into EH therapy. While some of these may be more structured or "techniqueish" than EH typically prefers, others fit more fluidly with EH approaches. Even more structured approaches can be a valuable integrative strategy. These and other EH approaches seek to help clients clarify and connect with meaning in their lives. Vos and Vitali (2018) found phenomenological and experiential approaches to meaning to be particularly effective, which fits well with EH therapy's general framework.

Meaning has been found to be effective with a range of psychological difficulties, including hopelessness, anxiety, depression, and suicidal ideation (Vos, 2025a). Although there is limited research, meaning may also be important for people recovering from trauma, particularly when this involves an existential shattering or challenge to one's values or worldview. Meaning is useful in working with clients experiencing life transitions, particularly as they may be transitioning from one source of meaning to another.

Here-and-Now

Working with the here-and-now, also sometimes called immediacy, was first identified in Gestalt psychology (Krug et al., 2025); however, it has become a staple in humanistic and EH psychology. The here-and-now "refers to what is emerging, in the *here* of the therapy room and the *now* of the immediate moment" (Krug, 2009, p. 330). Krug distinguished between an intrapersonal and an interpersonal focus with the here-and-now. The intrapersonal approach focuses on what is happening within the client in the present moment, while the interpersonal focuses on what is emerging between the client and therapist in the present moment. Both are valuable and used by most EH therapists.

Here-and-now work involves inquiring about or calling attention to what is happening in the present moment. Inquiring may involve asking or being curious about what the client is experiencing in the moment. Calling it to attention can involve marking nonverbals, reflecting emotion, and using intuitions about what is happening. These are explored by the client and therapist together. One aspect of here-and-now work can involve the therapist's self-disclosure pertaining to their experience in the present moment. There are various reasons for such self-disclosures, as discussed in the Self-Disclosure section.

The use of the here-and-now has a strong empirical basis (Hill et al., 2018; Underwood, 2025). The here-and-now can be particularly helpful when interpersonal challenges are the presenting concern or are contributing to other difficulties, such as depression and anxiety. It is also associated more generally with improvements in mental health.

Self-Disclosure

There are various types of therapist self-disclosure and ways to approach self-disclosure (Sebree & Brown, 2025). One type of self-disclosure is immediacy, or self-disclosure in the moment with the client (i.e., here-and-now). This may include forms of encouragement, reinforcing the progress, and inviting the client to disagree with the therapist, which also includes the therapist sharing their reactions to the client in the moment. This facilitates a corrective relational experience, particularly when a client is expecting a negative reaction, such as punishment or rejection, based on past experiences. Sharing one's thoughts, feelings, or process in the moment models disclosure, encourages the client's genuineness, and facilitates the development of relational depth.

Another type of disclosure is personal disclosures, which include personal revelations about the therapist. This type of disclosure is strongly discouraged in many, if not most, therapy modalities and in some clinical contexts or settings. While there are important context considerations, such as working in a prison or with clients struggling with certain types of boundary issues, personal self-disclosure can be beneficial in modeling for clients, providing hope, and building relational depth. However, it is crucial that disclosures are done thoughtfully and for the benefit of the client. At times, these benefits may be indirect, such as through deepening the relationship, while at other times, they may be direct, such as providing hope or modeling for the client. Personal self-disclosures should generally be brief, and caution should be used to ensure that it does not shift the focus of therapy to the therapist.

The client's culture and previous experiences should be considered with self-disclosure (see Sebree & Brown, 2025). In some cultures, self-disclosure may be experienced differently and signify different meanings. In addition, prior experiences, such as boundary crossings by previous therapists or authority figures, impact how clients experience the therapist's disclosure. In addition to considering these factors before self-disclosures are made, especially personal self-disclosures, EH therapists should closely observe how clients respond to the therapist more generally and their openness in therapy.

As illustrated, different types of disclosure may serve different purposes, and disclosures contribute to either direct or indirect benefits. Self-disclosure may be particularly beneficial for clients struggling with certain relational difficulties. It may also be beneficial for individuals with anxiety, particularly social anxiety, and issues such as loneliness, isolation, and alienation, which often are connected to depression. Sebree and Brown (2025), in their review of the research on self-disclosure, noted that increasing the frequency of self-disclosure often led to an improved therapy relationship and decreased symptomology.

Positive Regard and Acceptance

Positive regard or acceptance is an intervention that is often misunderstood or misrepresented. For example, this is often understood as the therapist accepting or approving of all the client's choices or behaviors, a rather shallow or weak understanding of acceptance. Rather, acceptance refers to accepting the person of the client, including their mistakes, errors, shortcomings, and other flaws, which often changes how one understands or experiences these (see Hoffman et al., 2013). There is a cyclical process that often occurs with acceptance. The client's experience of the therapist's acceptance encourages them to disclose more, including what they perceive as more risky disclosures. From the foundation of acceptance of the person of the client, the therapist can seek a deeper understanding of what brought about the problematic behavior. As they do this, it becomes more difficult to judge the client, which leads to a deeper acceptance of them. It is not condoning the behavior but empathetically understanding and not judging as clarity emerges as to why they behaved the way they did. This acceptance facilitates many potential benefits, including greater relational depth, the client's forgiveness of themselves, the client's self-acceptance, and the client's continued disclosure.

For acceptance or positive regard to be effective, it must be communicated. While this can be communicated directly, such as voicing one's acceptance of the client, it is more powerful when demonstrated through the therapist's behavior and responses to clients. Many clients have told us that they know we accept them even without us voicing acceptance. This is a powerful form of acceptance; however, it is bolstered by finding ways to voice this genuinely.

Acceptance, like many of the interventions we have discussed, has direct and indirect benefits. The indirect benefits include strengthening the therapeutic alliance, promoting relational depth, and encouraging self-disclosure. The direct benefits include contributing to a corrective relational experience and facilitating the client's self-acceptance. These can be helpful for clients with excessive self-criticalness, anxiety, depression, and various forms of interpersonal difficulties, including loneliness and trust issues.

Using Objective or Guiding Stances and Psychoeducation

While EH therapy is known for its focus on the subjective experience of the client, Bugental (1987, 1999) and May (1958) both advocated a place for objectivity as well. Subjectivity and objectivity are understood as part of a dialectical process. EH therapy's concern has been the excessive reliance on or idealization of objectivity in which the client's subjective experience or perspective is devalued or dismissed. Generally, strategies rooted in objectivity are used sparingly and situationally. There are situations, such as when a client presents as a danger to themselves or others, when it is important to use a more objective perspective, including assessing for safety. At times, this may even include using objective assessment measures. Similarly, when clients experience extreme states, including those associated with severe psychiatric diagnoses, using an objective stance is needed, even if it is balanced with trying to understand the client's subjective experience.

Helping clients engage in a dialectical process with subjectivity and objectivity can help them clarify their subjective experience. This can be engaged through shifting between different stances with the client and using a searching process that encourages self-reflection. Similarly, encouraging clients to consider objective and empathetic perspectives can help them better understand people with whom they experience conflict. Here, again, the objective perspective is considered in a dialectic, this time with empathy.

EH approaches tend to emphasize following the client, not guiding. However, again, there are times when guiding the client is valuable or necessary. For example, the therapist may, at times, guide the client to consider particular topics or perspectives. Similarly, therapists may need to direct attention to a theme, issue, or concern. Again, these are typically used sparingly. Psychoeducation can be a form of guiding the client as well. It helps the client consider a particular perspective, which may include research, theoretical perspectives, or other sources of information. Typically, when EH therapists employ psychoeducation, it is with an emphasis on the client considering different perspectives, not suggesting them as truth, answers, or solutions. It is beneficial to make this explicit to avoid imposing values, interpretations, or direction on clients.

We hesitated to include these interventions, particularly because they are used infrequently and sparingly. However, because research has indicated that EH therapists have identified these as commonly used (see Hoffman & Cleare-Hoffman, 2017a), it is important to include them. We want to emphasize, however, that a primary concern from an EH perspective is making sure these do not shift the frame away from being primarily focused on the client's experience and direction.

Integrative Strategies

A variety of integrative strategies can be used in EH therapy (see Schneider, 2007). Any purist approach has significant limitations. The challenge is striving to integrate them consistently. We recommend a critical assimilative approach to integration (see Schneider et al., in press) that seeks to integrate strategies to ensure what is integrated is consistent with the foundation. For example, Hoffman (2021) recommended, "When integrating with an existential–humanistic foundation, it is important to consider which strategies are consistent with its underlying philosophy and values. At times, strategies that are integrated require modification to fit with the existential–humanistic foundation" (p. 40). The addition of "critical" is important as it embodies an openness to engaging in critical reflection about the assimilative integration, including, if needed, making adjustments to the EH approach. This is crucial when considering multicultural perspectives. If EH therapy is only willing to integrate multicultural frameworks when they fit or are modified to fit with the EH foundation, it is not truly integrating multicultural perspectives. EH must be willing to change, too, if it becomes apparent this is needed or beneficial for clients. This balances the need for a consistent foundation with true openness.

It is not realistic to consider all the possible integrations with EH therapy in a chapter or even a book. In the following sections, we consider select interventions that fit closely with EH therapy. In addition, some EH therapists may advocate that these are part of EH proper, not just interventions that could more readily be integrated into EH therapy with minimal concern about how they fit with its foundation.

Experiential Techniques

EH therapy is sometimes described as an experiential therapy (see Schneider, 1998). Watson and colleagues (1998) defined experiential therapy, stating, "The main objective of experiential therapy is working with clients' awareness, both by focusing on subjective experience and by promoting reflexivity and a sense of agency" (p. 3). Experiential techniques, then, are more structured interventions intended to accomplish this, such as empty- or two-chair techniques and emotion-focused, Gestalt, and somatic interventions (Cole, 2025). These techniques are used to stimulate and sometimes release emotion. The activation of emotion is combined with reflection. Experiential techniques are particularly useful when working with emotions and facilitating self-awareness. Therefore, they often are integrated with the primary EH intervention strategies discussed previously.

Creative and Expressive Arts Interventions

The creative and expressive arts are closely connected with EH therapy, and some, arguably, emerged from EH psychology (see Serlin et al., 2025). The creative arts therapies include poetry, painting, dance, journaling, and more. At times, the client engages in these through reading or observing, while at other times, clients write or participate in these interventions. Like the experiential techniques, these are often used to stimulate and process emotions while also encouraging reflection. Also, like experiential techniques, they can be particularly useful with emotional processing and promoting self-awareness. They provide a release or processing of emotion at the bodily or somatic level.

Mindfulness

Mindfulness has become one of the most popular interventions in contemporary therapy; however, there is controversy about mindfulness. The term mindfulness is derived from Buddhism, and mindfulness techniques are generally drawn from Buddhism; however, when mindfulness is implemented in therapy, it is generally done to pursue different outcomes (Hoffman et al., 2020). Mindfulness in Buddhism is not primarily used for mental health benefits;

however, in therapy, the focus is almost always on the acceptance and management of emotions with the goal of improved mental health. In many Buddhist approaches, mental health benefits are a side effect, not the primary objective. In other words, mindfulness has been appropriated from Buddhism and changed without acknowledging this or seeking consent. While it could be argued that psychology should use a different name than mindfulness to show respect to Buddhism, the reality is that mindfulness is here to stay. It has been too thoroughly appropriated to be easily changed.

What is called mindfulness in therapy today is not significantly different from treatment strategies that have been common in EH therapy long before mindfulness was popularly incorporated into therapy. As such, whether integrating mindfulness strategies adds anything new to EH therapy can be questioned. EH therapy has long encouraged clients to engage in nonjudgmental reflection, including emotional, somatic, and bodily awareness, through focused attention to one's thoughts and body. Integrating mindfulness may be adding a new name for what EH has long been doing instead of adding new strategies; however, it may introduce new, creative strategies as well that can be incorporated in pursuit of nonjudgmental awareness. For example, mindfulness interventions often include guided or structured processes that engage clients in reflection, which can sometimes be helpful. Mindfulness and similar EH strategies can be useful in promoting self-awareness, working with emotions, vivifying resistance, engaging the here-and-now, and promoting self-acceptance.

CONCLUSION

In this chapter, we provided an overview of the primary EH intervention strategies identified through research with EH therapists and reviewed influential overviews of EH therapy. The intervention strategies were briefly introduced; however, it is important to recognize that these are complex interventions, and it often takes years to develop competency in implementing them. A brief overview, such as provided in this chapter, may give the false impression that these are rather simple strategies that are easy to implement and master. However, as students generally recognize when beginning to implement these treatment strategies, they are far from simple, and it takes training, supervision, and practice to learn to use them effectively.

A primary limitation that must be considered when implementing these interventions is the need to modify them according to individual and cultural differences. Most of these interventions are covered in greater depth in *The Evidence-Based Foundations of Existential–Humanistic Therapy* edited by Hoffman and Lac (2025). Each of these chapters provides (a) an overview of the intervention, (b) a review of the empirical research on the intervention, and (c) considerations of how these interventions may need to be adapted for work with individuals from different cultural backgrounds.

Our intent in this chapter was to cover these approaches sufficiently enough to provide a guide for the treatment planning section. Therefore, with each intervention, we included a brief overview, a couple of considerations of how to implement the intervention, and consideration of the issues and/or concerns for which these interventions may be particularly useful. As it was not realistic to provide a more comprehensive overview and examples of how to implement these treatment strategies, a list of recommended readings to deepen one's understanding of these interventions and strategies is included in Appendix B. This chapter gives a taste of the interventions. We hope readers who are not familiar with these strategies have developed a hunger to delve deeper.

3

Case Example Introduction

Rasheeda

In this chapter, we introduce a client who is followed through the next several chapters, illustrating how to fill in the case formulation. A challenge is that the case formulation is intended to be fluid. Therefore, for some sections, particularly the case formulation, two versions are included: one after eight sessions and one after 30 sessions. In this introduction, the final 10 sessions are also included. Although the final 10 sessions are not updated in the case formulation, they are included to illustrate how moving toward the end of therapy can lead to new issues emerging.

The client, Rasheeda, is fictionalized. We strove to make the case realistic, often inspired by common themes and types of interactions that we have had with our clients. While some aspects of the therapy process are discussed, the purpose of the case is primarily to illustrate how to do an existential–humanistic (EH) case formulation rather than EH therapy. Some discussion of the therapy process is included to illustrate changes between the first version (through the first eight sessions) and the second version (through the first 30 sessions). In this chapter, a thorough narrative of Rasheeda is provided. To avoid excessive repetition, aspects of Rasheeda's history are introduced in later sections, particularly the opening client narrative.

https://doi.org/10.1037/0000464-004
Case Formulation in Existential–Humanistic Therapy, by L. Hoffman and H. P. Cleare-Hoffman

INTRODUCING RASHEEDA

Rasheeda is a 33-year-old cisgender, multiracial woman who identifies as bisexual. Rasheeda's father was Black and was born in Alabama, though his parents moved to Colorado when he was 8 years old due to the pervasive racism he and his siblings experienced in school. Rasheeda's mother was born in India and immigrated to the United States when she was 2. Rasheeda reported that her parents had a good marriage, though there was often conflict between her parents and her grandparents, resulting in her not being close to any of her grandparents.

Rasheeda is the oldest of four children, with one sister, Maryam, and two brothers, Rohan and Jamar. She reported a good relationship with her siblings; however, the older brother, Rohan, has had a difficult life, resulting in Rasheeda often having to help him. Rasheeda reported a happy home life growing up. She stated, "Our whole family struggled with fitting in, including my parents and siblings. We bonded together to support each other when feeling isolated and lonely." Her father was patient at home with his wife and children, but Rasheeda knew that he could "have a bad temper outside of the family." Although her father had a master's degree, he had trouble maintaining consistent employment. Rasheeda reported that her father lost several jobs due to standing up to racism in the workplace, and eventually, he had trouble finding new employment because of this pattern.

At home, Rasheeda's father was patient, attentive, and always there to listen. However, he encouraged her to "be a strong woman," telling her that she had to be strong to survive. Rasheeda felt safe to come to her father with anything, saying, "He was my first therapist. He always listened, cared, and gave me good advice." Part of this advice was not to show any emotions outside her immediate family. Because of this, Rasheeda described herself as "feeling like a different person at home" compared with at school. She also reported that she got her sense of humor from her father. He loved to laugh and make his children laugh.

Rasheeda described her mother as "stable, hardworking, and serious." She was working to finish her teaching degree when Rasheeda was born. Due to financial constraints, she dropped out of college and began working as an administrative assistant for a real estate firm. Rasheeda's father always encouraged her mother to go back and finish her degree, but she insisted that they needed the stable income and health care benefits she received at her job. Rasheeda's mother showed little emotion, even to her husband and children. While Rasheeda reported a good relationship with her mother, she noted that she was not as close and "could not talk to her about anything emotional." She said only her father could get her mother to laugh and have fun. When her father was not around, her mother was always serious. When her father was between jobs, Rasheeda's mother would take on more hours at work and sometimes a second job. She reported that "this killed my father."

Rasheeda was close with her sister, who was 2 years younger. They shared many interests, including painting, poetry, reading, and hiking. She stated that only her father could make her laugh more than her sister. Growing up, both sisters did not have many friends, so they became each other's best friends. Her brothers were 5 and 7 years younger than her. The older brother, Rohan, was a good athlete and was involved in sports throughout high school and college, but he never took his grades seriously. Rasheeda loved watching him play soccer and baseball, describing herself as one of his biggest fans. Because of Rohan's involvement with sports, he had more friends than the rest of the family, but these did not seem to last as he grew older. He did not complete his coursework when his scholarship ran out and then dropped out of college. He moved frequently between jobs, either getting fired or quitting for "pitiful reasons." Her youngest brother, Jamar, was shy and studious. He was not involved with sports and did not have friends for most of his childhood and even adulthood. He graduated from college in 3 years and obtained his master's degree afterward. She reported loving him but not feeling as close because he isolated himself and focused on school and, later, work. Because Rasheeda's parents both worked, except when her father was between jobs, she took on a lot of responsibility for raising her brothers.

Growing up, Rasheeda loved school. She had a few friends, but none with whom she felt close. She went to a nearby college so she could live at home and commute to save money. This also allowed her to continue helping raise her brothers. She obtained her bachelor's degree at age 22 and master's degree in English literature at age 24, then taught high school English for 2 years before obtaining a job at a community college. At age 28, she started taking courses part time toward a Master of Fine Arts (MFA) in creative writing, which she reported was her "true passion."

While in college, Rasheeda met Edward, and they began dating. She had only been in a couple of short-term dating relationships before, mostly with women. She knew her mother never approved of her dating women, but she never said anything. Her father and siblings were more accepting. Edward was her first long-term relationship. He was smart, driven, and successful. Their relationship progressed quickly. When she introduced Edward to her family, her mother seemed pleased that she was dating "a successful White man from a good family." Her father, however, did not like Edward and let Rasheeda know. He told her he did not like how Edward treated her and that she could do better. Her father felt Edward expected her to cater to him and conform, and she readily obliged. He also worried that Edward was too serious.

During her final semester in her undergraduate program, Rasheeda's father became ill. The doctors had difficulty diagnosing what was wrong, but his health deteriorated quickly. Right before one of her midterm exams, she received a call from her mother, who said she had to come home immediately but would not tell her why. Rasheeda was upset, insisting that she had to take her exam. She did not obey her mother's demands and took her exam. When she arrived home after the exam, she found out that her father was dead. Rasheeda was heartbroken and filled with grief. While her family bonded together in the aftermath of her father's death, she sensed that her mother and sister were both angry at her for not coming home sooner. Her relationship with her sister did not feel the same for many years, though her sister denied that anything was different. As her father and sister were the only two she felt she could be emotionally vulnerable with, Rasheeda withdrew into herself and began bottling up her emotions. This was easy to do with Edward, who seemed to prefer this. Several weeks after her father's death, Edward proposed, and Rasheeda accepted.

Edward and Rasheeda set a wedding date for the summer after graduation. It was difficult for her not to have her father present, but she did not talk about this with anyone. After the wedding, Rasheeda insisted that they find a place to live within a few minutes of her mother's house so she could help with her brothers, who were still in high school. Because Rasheeda rarely insisted on anything, Edward agreed but soon became resentful of Rasheeda spending so much time helping her mother and brothers. Edward's family, too, became critical of Rasheeda. She felt increasingly alienated.

Rasheeda had always wanted children, but Edward refused to consider having children until Rasheeda was not so involved with her family. By the time her youngest brother graduated, Edward and Rasheeda were "disagreeing" regularly. Edward was not home most evenings, saying that he was working late. However, after a few months of this, a friend of Edward's, who Rasheeda had always liked, asked to stop by their home. He told her that Edward had been having an affair. Rasheeda did not respond with any emotions. When Edward arrived home, she calmly told him that she knew and asked him to go to marital therapy. Edward immediately countered, saying he wanted a divorce. He packed his bags that same evening and went to a hotel. The next week, he moved out with no further discussion.

Rasheeda was about to turn 29 years old and continued teaching at the community college after the divorce. She began to immerse herself in work and take more classes in her MFA program, where she met and became infatuated with a cisgender White woman named Spring. Rasheeda and Spring began dating. Their relationship quickly became intense. Rasheeda told Spring she was in love with her just under 2 months into the relationship. Spring responded, saying she was not interested in a committed relationship and abruptly ended the relationship. Rasheeda was upset. Over the next year and a half, she kept contacting Spring, begging her to change her mind. Spring was compassionate and understanding but kept telling Rasheeda she was not interested in anything more than friendship. Since her father's death, Rasheeda had only expressed her emotions with Spring.

Now 31, Rasheeda began fearing that she would never have a family. She tried dating both men and women, finally deciding that she wanted to focus on relationships with men in hopes of having a family with biological children. She described her world as "becoming smaller." Since her father's death, her life had become about work; Edward and, later, Spring; and then trying to find a new romantic partner. She took no vacations, did not go on hikes, stopped writing, and even stopped reading. She also withdrew from her family.

As her 33rd birthday approached, Rasheeda's sister began reaching out. At first, Rasheeda kept putting off talking to her. Finally, her sister stopped by the house, and they had a long conversation. Rasheeda shared that she felt her sister was mad at her because Rasheeda did not come home sooner when her father died. This time, her sister acknowledged this was true. They both shared openly with each other, crying and offering forgiveness.

Rasheeda and her sister began spending more time together, but Rasheeda still did not share much about what was happening in her life. Rasheeda's sister suggested a girls' weekend at a resort in the mountains, and she agreed. While they were away, Rasheeda's sister, now married, told Rasheeda she was pregnant. Though trying to feign excitement for her, her sister knew it was not genuine. She confronted Rasheeda on this, and Rasheeda denied it. However, that night, her sister heard her crying in her room and went in. This time, Rasheeda shared everything that had happened with Edward, Spring, and her life since her father's death. Her sister listened attentively and held her while she cried. The next day, Rasheeda's sister began encouraging her to find a therapist. Initially, Rasheeda strongly resisted. Her sister shared that she went to a psychologist after their father's death, and it helped. Rasheeda eventually agreed.

RASHEEDA'S FIRST EIGHT SESSIONS

The first eight sessions prioritized establishing a strong therapeutic alliance, clarifying presenting issues and goals, and beginning engaging the therapeutic process. With EH therapy, the early sessions balance establishing the relationship and orienting the client to the therapeutic process, developing curiosity, facilitating self-awareness, and instilling hope.

Session 1: Getting to Know Each Other and Assessing Goodness of Fit

Rasheeda entered the room for her first session quietly with a polite smile, asking, "Where should I sit?" Dr. H. responded, saying, "I usually sit in this chair. You can sit anywhere else you like." After looking at the seating options, she chose the chair closest to the door—the one seat that no client had previously selected for individual psychotherapy. Dr. H began, "Tell me what brings you here today?"

RASHEEDA: Well, to be honest, my sister convinced me to come.

DR. H: She was concerned about something.

RASHEEDA: Yes, well, a few things. A lot has happened over the last 5 years.

DR. H: [*Sensing her hesitancy*] It is hard to talk about what happened. [*Dr. H paused for 5 seconds, then seeing Rasheeda's discomfort, continued.*] Maybe you can start by telling me what has happened in the last several years, and we can go from there. Take your time.

RASHEEDA: About 4 years ago, my husband left me. It wasn't a good marriage anyway. But . . . I don't know . . . I just . . . it goes back further. I don't know.

DR. H: It's okay, Rasheeda. I can see this is hard for you. Is there something I can do to help you get started?

RASHEEDA: Well, my father always stressed that personal things are for family. [*Rasheeda's eyes showed a glimmer of tears as she mentioned her father.*]

DR. H: Your father—he's no longer here?

RASHEEDA: Yes. [*Rasheeda tried to rein in the emotions; she turned away from Dr. H and looked anxiously at the door.*]

DR. H: It's okay. We can get to that when you are ready. It's hard to share because you don't know me. I am not family, not even a close friend.

RASHEEDA: Yes.

DR. H: Okay, what would be helpful to know?

With Dr. H's question, Rasheeda appeared to relax slightly. At first, she asked a few questions about Dr. H's training, then a few more personal questions, including his marital status, children, if he liked to hike, and if he had worked with biracial people. Dr. H answered briefly but openly, including sharing that he was in a biracial family, too. With each question, it seemed Rasheeda became more relaxed and began sharing. As she shared, she remained composed. If she began tearing up, she would quickly attempt to rein it in before continuing. In the first session, she shared briefly about her father's death and the distance that emerged with her mother and sister. She moved through this quickly. Although Dr. H would often slow clients down and pursue more depth, recognizing that Rasheeda was not ready, he allowed her to move through this quickly for now. She spent more time on her marriage, divorce, and relationship with Spring. After about 40 minutes, Dr. H interjected.

DR. H: I appreciate you sharing with me. I know it was not easy. After hearing some of your story, I am confident we can make progress on the issues you mentioned. In the first session, I generally like to share a bit about my approach to therapy to see if it is a good fit for you. We have about 10 minutes left. Would it be okay if I shared some about my approach with you?

RASHEEDA: Yes.

Rasheeda was attentive and focused as Dr. H shared his approach to therapy. As he concluded, he asked Rasheeda if she had any questions. She paused reflectively for several seconds before saying that she had no questions at that time. When Dr. H asked, she affirmed that she would like to give psychotherapy with Dr. H a try.

Sessions 2 to 5: Building the Therapeutic Alliance, Developing Curiosity, and Facilitating Emotional Processing

Over the next several sessions (Sessions 2–5), Dr. H prioritized building a good therapeutic alliance using warmth, empathy, and genuineness. He continued intentionally using some brief personal self-disclosures each session, which were effective in solidifying the therapeutic relationship. Rasheeda appeared increasingly comfortable disclosing information, including increasingly personal information; however, she remained cautious with emotions. When emotions emerged in the here-and-now, she quickly moved away from them, often changing topics. Dr. H commented on this, but Rasheeda dismissed it, saying she did not like expressing emotions. Dr. H also used a couple of here-and-now disclosures about his reaction to what was happening in the therapy room, which Rasheeda seemed to reflect on briefly but quickly moved away from; she responded better to the personal disclosures. She continued to avoid any discussions of her parents and siblings. The focus remained mostly on her marriage, her relationship with Spring, and her desire for a family. The strongest emotions that came up in these first sessions were when she discussed feeling as if time was quickly running out on having a family of her own. This topic elicited anxiety and sadness that she would stay with for a few seconds, longer than with other emotions. In Session 5, Dr. H shifted the focus to obtain an emotional history.

DR. H: I often find it helpful to get a sense of how emotions were expressed in your family. Would you be okay with this?

RASHEEDA: I guess so.

DR. H: You guess?

RASHEEDA: Yes, it is okay.

With some focused questions and reflections for clarification, Rasheeda explained that both her parents showed few negative emotions at home but were much freer with pleasant emotions. Her father was much freer and more expressive with emotions than her mother. At times, she would hear her father get more animated with anger when talking with her mother about situations at work, but the anger was never directed at her mother. She heard her mother discussing her father's temper at work but never witnessed this directly. Her mother was the disciplinarian and, at times, would get angry at Rasheeda and her siblings, but the most that would happen was her raising her voice. Rasheeda did not see her maternal grandparents often, but when she did, they also were restrictive with emotions. Her paternal grandparents were "the most animated of all my family members."

With her siblings, she was freer to express emotions with Maryam. With her brothers, she modeled her emotions after her parents, often being careful in what she expressed. When taking care of her brothers, she sometimes expressed anger like her mother but only if her parents were not around. If she were ever to show anger with her parents around, they scolded her, regardless of who the anger was directed at. The message she derived from this is that anger is dangerous and should be avoided. This was reinforced by knowing that her father lost several jobs after getting upset when advocating for racial issues at work.

When Rasheeda was sad, her father and sister were her comforters. She felt safe revealing her fears, anxieties, and sadness with them. However, her father often reminded her to share emotions only with her family. If she talked about her sadness too long, her father would often say, "Okay, that's enough now." Rasheeda cautiously shared that she longed to be able to share her sadness with her mother, especially after her father's death, but her mother did not feel as warm and accepting. Her mother would provide brief comfort before telling Rasheeda to "straighten up and dry your tears." Because of her family's influence, she rarely shared emotions with friends.

RASHEEDA: I know I have not shown many emotions here, but it is far more than I share anywhere else, except sometimes with my sister.

DR. H: I get some mixed impressions as you say that. On the one hand, you seem proud that you have kept your emotions so contained. On the other hand, it also seems there is a longing to share your emotions more.

RASHEEDA: [*Pausing, appearing sad*] Maybe so. But nowhere is safe. Not anymore.

DR. H: Not since your father's death.

RASHEEDA: Yes.

DR. H: I hope that, with time, it will feel safe to bring them in here. Even though you have not shared much, when some emotion creeps in, I have felt a deeper connection between us. I appreciated that.

RASHEEDA: [*Pausing, with eyes watering a bit*] We'll see.

This showed some increased openness with emotions, but Dr. H recognized this was as much as Rasheeda was comfortable going into and honored that. As they continued with the emotional history, Rasheeda shared more about her marriage. She reported that, from early on, it was rare that warm or positive emotions were shared between her and Edward. Over the 7 years of their marriage, there were fewer and fewer emotions expressed. Rasheeda reported that Edward often appeared agitated but rarely raised his voice. She described his most common emotional expressions as "subtle anger" and "strictness."

Dr. H asked Rasheeda to explain "strictness" as an emotion. She said, "It is similar to anger but more controlled and intended to control me." Rasheeda described being afraid of this. When their marriage ended, she described this as an emotionless scene:

RASHEEDA: He came home, and I told him I knew about the affair. I suggested couples therapy. I know what you are thinking. Me suggesting couples therapy? [*Rasheeda smiled briefly, revealing the intended humor.*] I don't know if I really wanted to do it, but it seemed like the right thing to suggest. I never raised my voice or showed any sadness. It was all matter of fact. He responded in kind. He said that he did not want to go to marital therapy and, instead, wanted a divorce. There was no emotion in anything he said. The conversation lasted only a couple of minutes, then he went upstairs, packed a bag, and said I could reach him at a hotel if I needed anything.

DR. H: Just like a business transaction.

RASHEEDA: Exactly. It didn't feel like a marriage was ending, but maybe that was because it hadn't felt like a marriage for several years.

DR. H: Yet, there were some emotions.

RASHEEDA: I supposed there had to be some, right? But I don't remember feeling any . . . not for a while, at least. I know I felt something when it was final, but it was less about the marriage and more about just feeling alone. And wanting to move on. I started on dating apps the day the divorce was final and was on my first date within 2 weeks of it all being final.

DR. H: The emotions about the marriage just dissipated.

RASHEEDA: Yeah. [*Pausing*] Well, mostly. I did feel some shame and guilt. But this was more about me than Edward. Honestly, I think I was relieved he was out of my life. I felt some sadness earlier, months, even years, earlier. But nothing when it was actually over.

DR. H: Tell me about the shame and guilt.

RASHEEDA: [*Tearing up, then taking a breath*] It was my fault.

DR. H: The divorce?

RASHEEDA: No, the marriage. I never should have married him. My dad knew—he knew—Edward was not right for me. I should have listened. But I married him because . . . [*softly crying, then taking a breath*] I married him because I was alone. My dad was gone. My sister and mother were mad at me. I didn't share like that with my brothers. I needed someone, and Edward was there. There was nothing else special. He was just there—the wrong guy at the right time.

This was the longest that Rasheeda had stayed with emotions thus far. Still, it was less than a minute, but it showed some progress. We moved on to discussing her relationship with Spring. Rasheeda noted that her emotions were much freer with Spring, and she livened up when talking about her.

RASHEEDA: I was like a different person with Spring, freer with emotions than I had ever been. I still don't understand that. Was it that I had bottled things up as long as I could, and they just came bursting out? Or was it something about Spring that made me feel safe?

DR. H: Maybe both?

RASHEEDA: Probably.

DR. H: I am curious what that was like for you.

RASHEEDA: At times, it was exhilarating. I felt the most alive I had felt since . . . [*tears swelling up again*]

DR. H: Since your father's death.

RASHEEDA: [*Nodding while softly crying*]

The fifth session and the emotional history represented a transition in the relationship. Rasheeda gradually became more comfortable with emotions and emotional expression. It is important to emphasize that the focus is not on getting to emotions but moving into emotional processing. Bugental (1987) discussed emotional processing as entailing moving in and out of the emotion. While getting to emotion and facilitating emotional expression can be cathartic and useful, its utility is more limited if it is not accompanied by emotional processing, which includes sense making and meaning making. Part of the intent is to help clients become curious about their emotions (Hoffman, 2019c). The ability of many clients to stay with emotions in the here-and-now is an important reflection of the therapy relationship. With Rasheeda, it was increasingly clear that she longed for a safe place to express emotions, and therapy was slowly becoming such a space.

Rasheeda reported some work difficulties over the first five sessions as well. Although she was immersing herself in her job, her course evaluations had some items that disturbed her. In particular, her students reported that she seemed uninterested in the courses she was teaching and did not have time for their questions. Previously, her evaluations always viewed her as being engaged. Her department chair asked to speak with her and shared his concerns. He reported that she seemed increasingly withdrawn, missing meetings and no longer speaking in most meetings. When sharing this, Rasheeda commented, "I am working more—it seems almost all the time—but I am not being productive, or at least that's what my students and chair think." When Dr. H asked what she thought, after struggling a bit, she shared that she was embarrassed that it was difficult even to remember how she had been spending her time at work. After acknowledging this, she confirmed that she "must be disengaged."

Rasheeda also reported being more sensitive to feedback at work. When she first began teaching, Rasheeda was strongly offended and angered by some of the comments about her looks and clothing on course evaluations. The comments were often "complimentary" but personal and sometimes inappropriate. Over time, she still believed this was offensive but did not get upset about it and would skip over these comments. After her relationship with Spring ended, she became more upset by these comments again. While the inappropriate comments often appeared to be intended as positive, a couple noted that she put on weight and never smiled. Rasheeda was embarrassed about putting on almost 10 pounds in the months after the breakup with Spring. When Rasheeda received an "average" rating in her performance evaluation, she felt ashamed.

Early in her career, both when teaching high school and at community college, she experienced occasional microaggressive comments. Remembering her father's experience, she always brushed these off. In the last couple of years, she voiced being increasingly angry about the microaggressive comments. She never said anything in response but worried people could tell she was mad. She began ruminating about these thoughts, including fantasizing about how she would like to respond, knowing she never would. The ruminations about the microaggressions often kept her up at night with anxiety and anger.

Sessions 6 to 8: Deepening the Therapeutic Process

In Sessions 6 to 8, Rasheeda went into emotions more each week. The pace was slow and gradual but consistent. As she became more comfortable with her emotions, and Dr. H engaged them with acceptance and curiosity, Rasheeda, too, became more curious about them. This began shifting her experience of the emotions and helped her stay with them longer. It also empowered her to explore other difficult topics, but she still quickly moved away from her father's death. When Dr. H reflected on this, Rasheeda said she was not ready. Dr. H honored this.

An important emergent theme in Sessions 6 to 8 was Rasheeda's loneliness. This topic had come up before, but Rasheeda would not go far into it. Gradually, she began exploring more of her loneliness and recognized different aspects of it (aloneness, existential isolation, existential loneliness, and alienation, though she did not use those words). This led to explorations of what drew her to Edward and Spring at different points of her life.

RASHEEDA'S SESSIONS 9 TO 30

As the therapeutic alliance and trust deepen, therapy begins to shift. It allows for a transition to deeper engagement and work with emotions and self-awareness. The length of time for the shift to occur varies according to numerous factors, including trauma, prior experiences with therapy, and other relational factors.

Sessions 9 to 16: Engaging and Staying With Emotions and Deepening Self-Awareness

By Session 9, Rasheeda was engaging emotions in each session and stayed with them longer. In Sessions 9 to 15, Edward came up regularly, particularly her regret and shame about marrying him. As she clarified what drew her to him, both before and after her father's death, she became less hard on herself. In Session 15, she pronounced that she could not forgive herself for hurting herself and Edward. In subsequent sessions, when Edward was discussed, there was little emotion. This was different than her initial avoidance of emotion— now she had processed it instead of suppressing it.

Sessions 17 to 18: Processing a Sudden, Difficult Emotional Experience

Spring remained a central topic increasingly infused with emotion. Rasheeda often pronounced that she still loved Spring. She still pondered why Spring did not want to be with her and what she did wrong. In Session 17, Rasheeda entered the session disheveled, which she had never done before. She typically dressed nicely and was concerned about her presentation, which her mother always emphasized as important. On entering, she plopped down on the couch. In previous sessions, she had gradually moved away from the chair closest to the door, but this was her first time sitting on the couch. Dr. H remained quiet. Rasheeda shifted from her initial slouching position to sitting up; she leaned forward into her hands and began crying. Dr. H sat silently before speaking.

DR. H: Something happened.

RASHEEDA: Spring is engaged.

DR. H: Wow, I'm sorry, Rasheeda.

RASHEEDA: So, it was me, after all. She didn't want to be with me. It was all bull . . . it was all bullshit. She didn't choose me. It wasn't that she didn't want a committed relationship. She didn't want me.

This session marked a shift. When talking about Spring before, there was always a sense of hope that someday, Spring might be ready for a committed relationship and reach out to Rasheeda. Although Rasheeda had been dating occasionally over the last 2 years and had begun exclusively dating men, saying she was focusing on a family, she had not been on more than five dates. Dr. H wondered if this was because of Spring and gently explored how her relationship with Spring impacted her subsequent relationships, but Rasheeda always dismissed the relevance of Spring in new relationships. She had only been on two dates with the same man since returning to therapy.

Although he kept calling, Rasheeda kept putting off seeing him again, canceling several dates.

Spring was a common topic in therapy; however, Rasheeda always focused on why she was drawn to Spring, her sadness from the relationship ending, and her longing to be close to her again. She would never go too deep, despite encouragement from Dr. H. Now, Rasheeda started to go deeper.

DR. H: Spring was important to you. She was a good friend, and you cared deeply for her, but it seems she also represented something more.

RASHEEDA: Maybe so. I know you've tried to get me to look at this before. But I . . . [*her voice trails off before a few moments of silence*]

DR. H: You . . .

RASHEEDA: I didn't want to just analyze my relationship with her.

DR. H: It didn't feel right to talk about her that way.

RASHEEDA: No, it didn't. I mean, I loved her. She was not just a topic for therapy. She was someone I thought could be the love of my life.

DR. H: You were afraid that talking about her and why she was important would do something.

RASHEEDA: [*Pausing*] Yeah, I didn't want to find out that I didn't really love her.

DR. H: That seems significant. You were protecting something.

RASHEEDA: [*Tears welled up, then she looked to the window, which she often did when moving away from her emotions.*]

DR. H: Stay with that for a moment, Rasheeda. I think this may be important. Your tears are saying something.

RASHEEDA: It was different with her. I felt different; I felt freer.

DR. H: You were different.

RASHEEDA: I was different. [*Long pause*] I miss who I was with her.

Rasheeda had been going into her emotions more over the course of therapy, but in this session, she started going deeper with self-reflection. As she did this, she recognized and considered her choices more, including her choices in relationships.

In the next session, Session 18, Rasheeda continued to focus on Spring. She was able to move in and out of the emotion more readily; in the previous session, she quickly became overwhelmed with the emotion. In Sessions 17 and 18, she spent more time exploring how she was different with Spring, including when she would smile talking about times when they were more deeply connected.

DR. H: I'm noticing something today. Last week and today, I have felt more connected to you. I wonder if you've felt that, too.

RASHEEDA: [*Pausing to reflect*] I hadn't noticed, but I am feeling more comfortable in here. [*Pausing*] And, yes, part of that is feeling more connected.

DR. H: What do you think about that?

RASHEEDA: Well, I guess I'm being more honest with myself.

DR. H: That makes sense. And as you are more honest with yourself, it seems you are more honest and open in here.

RASHEEDA: Yeah, that seems to fit.

DR. H: With Spring, too, you were more open and honest—you revealed yourself more.

RASHEEDA: [*Tearing up*] Yeah . . . [*starting to cry more openly*]. It was the only time . . . [*having difficulty speaking because of crying*]. It was the only . . .

DR. H: It was the only time since your father's death.

RASHEEDA: [*Crying heavily*]

This recognition was important for Rasheeda and led to increased awareness of how the ways that she engages in relationships contributed to her feeling isolated, lonely, and, at times, alienated. After this session, she began talking about her father more, including moving into grief and his death, as well as grief about the lost years of connection with her sister and her continued feelings of disconnection with her mother. Dr. H began wondering about the idealization of her father, along with a need to protect him. Recognizing the protectiveness, Dr. H tagged this for later but did not explore it.

Beginning with Session 18, Rasheeda's work in the here-and-now shifted. The dialogue from Session 18 represented the first time she engaged in the here-and-now interpersonally. She increasingly engaged in the here-and-now intrapersonally with her own emotions but avoided interpersonal here-and-now explorations pertaining to the therapy relationship.

Sessions 19 to 25: Processing Grief Over Rasheeda's Father and Feelings of Loneliness and Isolation

After a few sessions focusing primarily on grief with Spring and her father, with a gradual shift to being more focused on her father, Dr. H recognized an opportunity to explore the possible idealization and protectiveness of her father.

RASHEEDA: [*Pausing before speaking*] There were times when my father told me to shut down my emotions, but it was always after being there for me. I could cry with him and my sister, but never for too long. He was my go-to person.

DR. H: It is evident that you loved and trusted your father. I am hearing that your father felt safe and that you could open up your emotions with him. And I am also hearing that, at times, you had to push them back down.

RASHEEDA: [*With a somewhat defensive tone*] Yeah, but he knew what he was doing. He was protecting me. He knew from his own experience that it was not safe to share emotions out in the world. He was doing what was best.

DR. H: I can see that. I am also hearing you talk about how this may have contributed to you pushing down a lot of emotions in other places.

RASHEEDA: It wasn't his fault. It isn't always safe out there. He did what he needed to do to protect me.

DR. H: It seems you feel you need to defend your father.

RASHEEDA: Yeah! I don't know why you are going after him today. He was a great father! [*Tears welling up*]

DR. H: He was. I wish I could have met him.

RASHEEDA: [*Still crying*] Then why are you criticizing him?

DR. H: I'm not intending to criticize him. I can tell he was a great father and that you loved him very much. But even great fathers doing their best may do some things that lead to us getting hurt.

RASHEEDA: He never hurt me! He would never have done that!

DR. H: I am not saying he hurt you, but his attempts to protect you from the world also ended up contributing to you feeling isolated. He didn't intend that, but it was a side effect of sorts.

RASHEEDA: [*After a long silence*] But he didn't . . .

DR. H: He didn't what?

RASHEEDA: He didn't hurt me. He didn't want me to be alone.

DR. H: No, he didn't. He loved you and wanted what was best for you. He shared what he had learned to protect himself, just like you have to decide how you want to be in the world.

Through dialogues such as this, Rasheeda felt less of a need to protect her father, and gradually, her idealization of him lessened. She still thought he was a great father—and he was—but he was not perfect, as no father is. In processing her emotions about her father, she began to recognize her relationship choices, including keeping her emotions out of most relationships. As this occurred, her feelings of loneliness and isolation became more prominent in Sessions 20 to 25.

RASHEEDA: I am just so lonely all the time. I mean, except when I am with my sister, but she is getting ready for her daughter to be born. She has other things to focus on, so I don't want to take up too much of her time, especially with my problems. So, I am just left feeling alone. I mean, I still see her each week and talk to her most days. I enjoy this. But it isn't enough.

DR. H: You want other relationships where you don't feel alone.

RASHEEDA: Yeah. I try once in a while with my mother, but it is so obvious that I cannot talk to her. Rohan has enough problems of his own. It seems with him, I am just helping him. And Jamar, well, Jamar seems like he is doing great, at least professionally, but we still just don't connect.

DR. H: And in here?

RASHEEDA: I feel connected in here. But sometimes it feels like you are my best friend—my only friend.

DR. H: There is something different in here.

RASHEEDA: Yeah, you listen, and I can tell you care. I can be myself in here.

DR. H: I've appreciated that. Over the last several months, it does seem you are being yourself in here more, and I feel more connected to you as a result.

RASHEEDA: It is nice. At first, I think I was trying too hard to control how you saw me. I only shared what felt safe.

DR. H: And now?

RASHEEDA: It feels safe to share pretty much anything.

DR. H: You don't have that in relationships outside of here, but you want that.

In this exchange, Rasheeda continued to deepen her recognition of how she contributed to her experience of isolation. Gradually, she began considering, then implementing, taking more chances with a couple of friends. Some went well, while others she recognized were not people with whom she would want to pursue a deeper relationship. Early in therapy, she stopped dating after the two dates with one man. Recently, she began dating again and talked about wanting to be different on her dates. She was still just dating men but had also begun talking with some women on dating apps. The conversations with women did not lead to any dates, but she was enjoying the conversations.

Sessions 26 to 30: Identifying, Disclosing, and Processing a Sexual Assault

In Session 26, Rasheeda seemed different. Dr. H marked this to himself but did not say anything. After the session, Dr. H realized that it had been the least productive session with Rasheeda since she began therapy. Session 27 started similarly. Dr. H decided to explore this about halfway through the session.

DR. H: Rasheeda, last session and this session so far has seemed different. We've not been getting into topics as deeply. I'm noticing, too, that I'm feeling disconnected, and I'm wondering if you are experiencing that, too.

RASHEEDA: Yes, I am. I'm preoccupied.

DR. H: Tell me about that.

RASHEEDA: There is something that I've been wanting to bring up. When we first started, I was determined that I would not talk about it—not ever. But now I know I need to, and I think I feel okay about bringing it up. But I keep chickening out.

DR. H: You think you feel okay to talk about it. Maybe we can start there.

RASHEEDA: Everything I have brought up here has been okay, so I have no reason to believe this wouldn't be.

DR. H: But something is holding you back. I wonder if you can get in touch with what is holding you back.

RASHEEDA: [*Pausing*] Yes, I can feel it right here [*pointing to her upper chest, just below her neck*].

DR. H: Stay with that a moment. It seems this is trying to tell you something.

RASHEEDA: That it is not safe. I know that feeling. It is telling me that it is not safe. But I know it is.

DR. H: Your body and your mind are not in agreement.[1]

RASHEEDA: No, they are not.

DR. H: Your body is trying to prevent your mind from saying something.

RASHEEDA: Yes, exactly.

DR. H: If you stay with that and inquire why your body feels it is unsafe, I am curious to hear what it tells you.

RASHEEDA: [*Pausing*] I think it goes back to my father again, at least partly— back to not sharing personal things.

DR. H: Go on.

---

[1]This is being used as a metaphor. EH theory does not ascribe to a mind–body dualism. It was discussed earlier in therapy that statements such as this are intended as metaphors.

RASHEEDA: But I am just ashamed [*eyes starting to glisten with tears*].

DR. H: This one is difficult; it feels different than other things you have disclosed.

RASHEEDA: Yes, but I know it is safe. We've been through this with my father. And you've never judged me for anything. I think it's time.

DR. H: It is up to you. We have about 20 minutes left today. It is up to you if you want to share today, if this feels like enough time, or if you want to reflect on it more.

RASHEEDA: I'm afraid that if I don't say it today, I will lose my courage.

DR. H: Okay.

RASHEEDA: After Edward and I separated, I went out for drinks with a man at work—another professor—a couple of times over a few weeks. He was a friend, or I thought he was. They weren't dates; we were just talking. I shared with him that I was getting a divorce but didn't go into details about it. One night, I had too much to drink, so he offered to give me a ride home. When we arrived at my place, he asked if he could use the bathroom. I said this was fine. That night, I felt an attraction to him that I had not before. I think it was the wine. When he came out of the bathroom, I gave him a look.

DR. H: A look?

RASHEEDA: Yeah, a look that, I think, revealed that I was attracted to him. I didn't want to act on it, or at least I don't think I did. He had been walking to the door but then came over and kissed me. It was a good kiss. Or at least it seemed like it, but I was a bit drunk, which was something that I never do. Then, I came to my senses and pulled back. I told him I couldn't, that I wasn't divorced yet, and we were colleagues. He told me not to worry about that and kissed me again. I pulled away, but he kept kissing me and started feeling my breasts. I knew he wanted it and quietly said "stop" a couple more times, but he kept going, and I stopped resisting. We had sex. By the time we were done, I was sobering up and felt so ashamed. I told him he better leave because my mother was just a few houses away. I didn't want her to see, and I just wanted him to go so that I could forget about it. I needed him to be out of my house. The next day at work, I couldn't look at him. He took the hint, and we have never spoken again except in meetings. I am so ashamed. I mean, I wasn't divorced yet, and here I am whoring around. I've never told anyone.

As Rasheeda told the story, she did not look at Dr. H, mostly staring at the floor off to the side of him. There was some emotion but more anxiousness than sadness. It was evident that she felt it was her fault and did not recognize that this was a sexual assault. She had asked him to stop multiple times, both verbally and by pulling away from him, but he persisted. It is not uncommon to wait to disclose something like this until further into therapy. Dr. H marked several changes and then, when there were enough markers across two sessions to suggest something was going on, began to reflect these to the client. He did not push Rasheeda to reveal anything but rather honored her pace. Had he pursued, there is a greater chance she would have moved away from revealing what occurred. However, as he remained gentle and presented an invitation to disclose, she felt increasingly safe and chose to take the risk.

Over the subsequent sessions, Rasheeda discussed feelings of guilt from having led him on and, in her mind, encouraging him. Gradually, she started to recognize that it was not her fault, leading her to recognize that it was a sexual assault. With this acknowledgment, her emotions began to shift. She still felt guilt and shame, but she also began feeling anger and sadness. Dr. H worked to honor all these emotions. Anger was particularly difficult for her, as Dr. H recognized.

DR. H: It is hard to stay with the anger, even in here.

RASHEEDA: I don't like anger. It doesn't feel safe.

DR. H: Tell me about that.

RASHEEDA: I just don't like how it feels. I worry, too, about what will happen if I get angry at work.

DR. H: That didn't work out well for your father when he got angry at work.

RASHEEDA: [*Starting to cry*] No, it didn't.

DR. H: That's part of it.

RASHEEDA: Yeah, but I also just don't like anger. I've never allowed myself to be angry before.

DR. H: There is something that may happen if you become angry.

RASHEEDA: I don't know. I don't know what will happen.

DR. H: That unknown is part of it.

RASHEEDA: I just can't be out of control.

DR. H: There's another piece. [*Rasheeda looks anxious and tense.*] I can see the tension as we talk about this. It is in your jaw and shoulders, and I'm guessing it is elsewhere, too.

RASHEEDA: I feel it everywhere.

DR. H: And if you let that tension go?

RASHEEDA: I don't know. I don't know if I would scream or cry, but I know something would happen. Something would come out.

DR. H: I won't ask you to let it go. Just stay with the tension a bit. See if you can hear anything else about what it is saying.

RASHEEDA: [*Pausing*] It is asking why you are pushing me.

DR. H: Okay, good, so it is telling me to back off.

RASHEEDA: Yeah, I think so.

DR. H: And what if you were to tell me this?

RASHEEDA: [*Looking up directly at Dr. H*] I couldn't do that. I wouldn't do that.

DR. H: That shift there is important—from couldn't to wouldn't.

RASHEEDA: I don't want to. I mean, it's scary to do that.

DR. H: It is okay; I can handle it. You can tell me to back off at any time. You are in charge of what we talk about and the pace with which we talk about it.

RASHEEDA: Now I don't feel like I need to tell you to back off.

DR. H: Go on.

RASHEEDA: You are just doing it.

DR. H: I'm respecting your boundaries.

After this exchange, Rasheeda began shifting her relationship with anger. She never became comfortable yelling or becoming viscerally or vocally upset, but she was able to use her anger creatively to set boundaries. Rasheeda was more open to recognizing her anger as well. Previously, when anger emerged, she avoided or suppressed it. Now, she began moving toward welcoming it and eventually was able to welcome it. As soon as she was aware of anger, she began finding creative ways to use it. At times, this would be calmly voicing her anger or frustration, while at other times, it was removing herself from the situation or setting boundaries.

When Rasheeda first accepted that she was sexually assaulted, she strongly stated that she could not report what occurred, going as far as stating that she was not capable of reporting it. Over time, this shifted to saying that people would not believe her, especially because the man who assaulted her was a popular professor. Dr. H secretly hoped she would file a complaint against him or report it to the police, but he recognized it was not his decision, and she never reported it. Eventually, however, she decided that it was important to do something. She decided to confront her colleague but wanted to do it the day before a session in case it went poorly. For additional support, Rasheeda also shared with Rohan what had happened before confronting her colleague.

He was empathetic and supportive but also angry. She asked him to go with her when she stopped by her colleague's office and succinctly said,

> I told my brother about what happened between us. It was wrong. He is here to support me. I spent a long time feeling ashamed and believing it was my fault, but I said no—repeatedly. You should have stopped when I told you to. I do not feel safe being around you, being in meetings with you, or serving on committees with you. I decided not to report what happened as long as I don't hear that you have ever done anything like this to anyone else and as long as you honor my boundaries. You should take the lead in avoiding being on committees with me. I should not have to say that I do not want to be on a committee with you. I don't want to have a conversation about this. I am working through it in my therapy, and I encourage you to do the same.

The colleague began to apologize, but Rasheeda cut him off, reminding him that she did not want to talk about it. After this, Rasheeda left. Rohan gave her a big hug and told her that he was proud of her. Their relationship continued to improve, which was good for both Rohan and Rasheeda. The next day, Rasheeda entered therapy smiling and said, "I did it!" Dr. H celebrated this with her. As they processed her experience of confronting her colleague, Rasheeda reported feeling a mixture of emotions but said the feeling of empowerment was beginning to overshadow the painful emotions. Rasheeda continued to process emotions related to the sexual assault in the coming weeks. Although she had brief periods of worrying something bad would happen because she had confronted her colleague, the negative feelings continued to decrease and feel more manageable.

Sessions 31 to 50: Continued Emotional Exploration, Self-Empowerment, and Social Connection

Rasheeda continued talking with Rohan and shared what happened with Jamar and Maryam. The four siblings began spending more time together and deepened their bond. She also became more open with her friends, though she did not share her sexual assault with anyone outside of her family until later in therapy. Rasheeda felt more empowered as she continued dating, which became more of a focus during Sessions 31 to 50. In Sessions 31 to 50, Rasheeda also began exploring how she wanted to respond to microaggressions at work and gradually started confronting these. She still experienced significant anxiety when addressing microaggressions, but she felt empowered by this, and her confidence in addressing them continued to grow.

RASHEEDA'S FINAL 10 SESSIONS

Around Session 51, Rasheeda and Dr. H began discussing her ending therapy. Rasheeda had renewed deep and rewarding relationships with her siblings and was getting along better with her mother. She felt more fulfilled at work and began engaging in more creative writing, including submitting a couple of short stories for publication, with one already accepted. In her dating life, she had been dating a man for several months, and the relationship was getting serious. He was the first person she dated with whom she shared openly about her marriage, relationship with Spring, and her sexual assault. He was empathetic and compassionate as she disclosed this information, which deepened their relationship. Rasheeda felt like she had accomplished what she desired and more in therapy. She also discussed this with her siblings, who shared how proud they were of her and agreed that she was doing much better. Dr. H and Rasheeda agreed that it was valuable to approach her graduation from therapy slowly over several weeks.

The week after they began discussing ending her therapy, Rasheeda reported increased anxiety and sadness, which surprised her.

RASHEEDA: [*Softly crying*] I guess I am not ready to begin working toward the end of therapy after all. I am back to where I was at the beginning. I've been crying all week, and here I am, crying again in session.

DR. H: Let's not rush to judgment and instead try to stay open to what is emerging. It is not my impression that you are back to where you were.

RASHEEDA: I am just sad and anxious, but I don't know why.

DR. H: Just stay with it. See where it takes you.

RASHEEDA: [*Pausing*] I've been thinking about my dad a lot again . . . and my mom.

DR. H: Tell me about that.

RASHEEDA: I just miss him [*softly crying*].

DR. H: I know, and I am guessing you will always have periods of missing him. He was a pretty great dad, and you loved him.

RASHEEDA: I thought this would be over now. I mean, we talked about him so much, and I thought it was better.

DR. H: Grief often reemerges, but as I sit with you, this feels different than before. I am curious if it feels different to you.

RASHEEDA: [*Reflecting*] Well, it does. I am not sure I can really describe it, but it doesn't seem as overwhelming.

DR. H: That seems like progress. You can be sad about your father without it overwhelming you.

RASHEEDA: I hadn't realized that.

DR. H: I wonder if its reemergence has anything to do with us approaching the end of therapy.

RASHEEDA: [*Starting to cry*] I hadn't considered that, but all these tears seem to be saying "yes."

DR. H: Tell me about that.

RASHEEDA: Part of me, well, most of me, thinks that I am ready. There's a whole 'nother part of me that doesn't want this to end, even if I am ready.

DR. H: It is hard. I will miss you, too. But stay with this a minute.

RASHEEDA: I am worried that it will all come back—all the sadness and anxiety and the darkness.

DR. H: That makes sense. Many people worry about that as we near the end of therapy. That is part of why it is beneficial to take it slowly. And it is normal to grieve for the end of the therapy relationship. I often grieve for clients when they are done with therapy, and I will grieve for the ending of our relationship.

RASHEEDA: Really? You'll grieve for me?

DR. H: Yes. I care about you, Rasheeda, and I have enjoyed working with you. I am sure I will continue to think about you at times and hope that you are doing well.

RASHEEDA: Wow, I thought you would just move on to your next client. That means a lot to me.

In the next couple of sessions, Rasheeda and Dr. H revisited grief with her father and briefly with Spring, too. They also focused on adjusting to life without therapy and reinforcing the changes she made. The fear of being on her own, without weekly therapy, emerged several times. Dr. H suggested they begin by tapering off the frequency of sessions, which Rasheeda agreed to. This helped. Although she reported missing the weekly sessions, it became easier after a couple of sessions with decreased frequency. Rasheeda also noticed she had less to talk about in sessions. And she noticed something new.

RASHEEDA: I have been thinking a lot more about my mother, and I often feel sad when I am thinking about her.

DR. H: Tell me more about that.

RASHEEDA: I mean, you know all this. We've always had a decent relationship, but we have not been as close as I was with my father and Maryam and now with Rohan and Jamar and even my boyfriend.

DR. H: You are very close with all your immediate family now except your mother.

RASHEEDA: I think that's it. It is more evident that we are not that close now.

DR. H: That seems important. Is there something you want to do with that?

RASHEEDA: Maybe it is time to start having some courageous conversations with Mom.

Rasheeda started spending more time with her mother over the next several weeks, including telling her mother that she was sad that they were not closer. Through these conversations, their relationship began to improve, but it was evident that it was not likely to ever be as close as Rasheeda's relationship with her father and siblings. In the next to last session, Rasheeda shared some concerns.

RASHEEDA: I guess I have some more grieving to do, huh?

DR. H: Sounds like it.

RASHEEDA: It sometimes gets wearisome. It feels like I am always grieving.

DR. H: How are you doing going into this round of grief? We have been talking about the next session being our last session. Do you feel we need to delay for a couple more sessions?

RASHEEDA: As much as I don't want coming here to end, I feel okay handling this on my own. But if it changes before next week, can we still delay it?

DR. H: Yes, of course. But I think you are on to something important here. It is best for us only to delay if you really feel you need it. It may still be tough to accept that your relationship with your mom may never be what you hoped it would be. But if you are able to manage it on your own, it may be a good start to handling this on your own.

Rasheeda agreed. The next session was the final session. Rasheeda shared some tears of appreciation and sadness in the last session—as did Dr. H.

4

Brief Holistic Client Narrative

This chapter reviews the first section of the case formulation template provided in Appendix A, in which the client's narrative is detailed and includes an example narrative following the case of Rasheeda from Chapter 3.[1] The opening client narrative may seem redundant; however, this is included to frame the overall case formulation holistically. When the case formulation approach has been used in training settings, this section most frequently has errors reflecting a general misunderstanding. This is likely because a narrative of this nature is unusual; therefore, few students or clinicians have written a narrative of this sort about their clients.

The opening narrative provides a framework that influences how the rest of the case formulation is viewed and interpreted. Opening client overviews are typically constructed according to the client's presenting issues or identified problems, often with initial etiological hypotheses and considerations. From an existential–humanistic (EH) perspective, it is important to begin with a more holistic view of the client that empowers the therapist and other providers or treatment team members who will read the document to see the client holistically. Therefore, the opening client narrative is intentionally not problem centered.

Constructing an opening narrative in this manner has a practical implication as well: To complete the case formulation, the therapist must be intentional about getting to know the client beyond their problem. This goes beyond the typical identification of client strengths, which is included as the opening

---

[1]Rasheeda is a fictionalized client inspired by common themes and types of interactions that we have had with our clients.

https://doi.org/10.1037/0000464-005
Case Formulation in Existential–Humanistic Therapy, by L. Hoffman and H. P. Cleare-Hoffman

subsection of the case formulation. When identified in a case formulation, client strengths are generally connected to the identified problem or are relevant to the presenting issues. While it is appropriate to include these, it is important not to focus just on client strengths relevant to clinical issues. If this becomes the focus, it narrows the therapist's perspective on the client.

The opening client narrative paints a holistic picture of the client apart from their presenting problem or concern. The presenting issue and related issues are addressed in subsequent sections. Therefore, it is important to avoid the temptation to digress into the problem. Once again, seeing the client in this manner brings an enduring change to how the therapist sees the client—urging the therapist to continue seeing the client as a whole person in context. In addition, it may help identify natural strengths and coping mechanisms that could easily be missed, even when identifying strengths. For example, Seely (2007), in addressing psychological responses to trauma, argued that structured interventions are often harmful because they interfere with the client's natural healing processes and coping mechanism (see also Jackson & Pintauro, 2026). Seely (2007) proposed that client-centered approaches, which facilitate the natural healing process, empower the client's natural coping mechanism, and follow the client's pacing, may be more effective for working with trauma. This is consistent with Bohart and Tallman's (1999) central argument in their book *How Clients Make Therapy Work*. The assumption that the therapist has the keys to what will heal the client may often interfere with natural processes. Instead, EH therapy prefers first to identify, support, and empower the client's natural ways of healing. When these are insufficient, therapists collaboratively help clients find appropriate alternatives.

To create a holistic picture of the client, the opening narrative includes the client's hobbies, values, dreams and aspirations, sources of meaning, successes, and important relationships. In addition, it should consider the client's social positions, such as their gender identity, cultural background, and spiritual or religious identity. Consideration should be given to sources of pride, past successes, past enjoyable experiences (e.g., vacations, accomplishments), and what clients like about themselves. It can consider how clients typically spend their day, the type of music they enjoy, and what television shows or music they like. The opening client narrative can include information on the activities they do with their friends and family, as well as activities they do on their own. What is specifically included should vary with the client. Many of these may serve as natural coping mechanisms or may be incorporated into coping mechanisms. For example, I (Louis) worked with a client who was a fan of Pink Floyd. He would often talk about their lyrics in session and, on several occasions, asked to listen to songs in session, to which I agreed. Over the course of treatment, I referred to themes he discussed in Pink Floyd's music that were relevant to what we were discussing. This increased the client's engagement and, on several occasions, led to insight. We also discussed ways he could incorporate music into coping when he felt overwhelmed. The preceding examples are not intended to be a checklist of information that should be gathered; rather, they reflect some possibilities of what may be included.

Generally, the opening narrative will be three to seven paragraphs, though it can be longer. As with all aspects of the case formulation, it is not necessary to obtain this information in the first session or even in the first three to five sessions. It can emerge over time. However, being attentive and interested in this content is important to introduce early in therapy because it impacts the therapy process. While it is also important not to allow this to take so much time that it distracts from focusing on the presenting concerns, discussing these topics and getting to know the client beyond their presenting issues is not just a distraction or detour from addressing the presenting issues. It is part of building a good therapy relationship and can inform aspects of therapy and the desired outcome. It also facilitates the development of relational depth.

Conversations about topics beyond the presenting issue provide other useful information that can be used in therapy. Getting to know a client's hobbies can help identify sources of meaning or interests. When a client is feeling overwhelmed, briefly shifting the focus of the conversation to a topic of interest can help them calm down. While distractions such as this, for good reason, often have a negative connotation in therapy, sometimes a brief distraction is effective in giving the client space from the intensity of feeling so that they can return and approach the emotion or topic more productively. In other words, it can serve as a natural coping mechanism (Seely, 2007). In addition, Seely (2007) noted that natural coping "involves periods of processing that alternate with periods of avoidance" (p. 176). Therefore, allowing for and even, at times, encouraging brief periods of distraction may facilitate a natural healing process in the client. Often, therapists view these distractions as resistance or avoidance, which they can be. Almost any healthy coping mechanism can be misused or used in the service of avoidance. However, EH therapists help clients use these more intentionally and evaluate when they are being used constructively or in the service of avoidance. Attending to the periods of distraction and active engagement can help identify the most effective pace for the client.

Another example helps clarify the value of distraction and getting to know the client beyond their presenting concerns. A client with an extensive trauma background often experienced mild to moderate dissociation in the first several sessions. Grounding techniques were minimally effective. In the first session, the client shared that he was an avid fan of dogs. In the next couple of sessions, the client began talking about his dog or asking questions about my dog when feeling overwhelmed. Through early recognition of this pattern, the client became more aware that he had developed this as a coping strategy. When he began dissociating, we briefly discussed dogs. At times, I introduced this by sharing a dog story or asking something about his dog. This helped the client return to being present in the moment. After this, I guided the client with a grounding exercise. Over time, the grounding activities became effective after briefer discussions of dogs and eventually no discussions about them. Gradually, the client had fewer dissociative experiences outside of therapy as well, and when he did, he was better able to manage them, sometimes through engaging with his dog. Over time, he used his relationship with me for grounding in therapy and his relationship with his dog for grounding at home. He could use the grounding exercises effectively, even though they were not effective when I tried to implement them earlier in therapy. From the beginning, the goal was to enable the client to manage intense emotional experiences with minimal or no dissociation or distraction. Integrating his interests into conversations helped accomplish this goal and deepened the conversation. It also helped him shift from unreflexively using distractions to using them intentionally. The intentional use decreased the overall frequency and reliance on distraction while bolstering his confidence to handle strong emotions or dissociations.

In the following illustration with Rasheeda, bolded text represents information that emerged later in therapy between Sessions 9 and 30. We recommend updating without bolding new material in an actual case formulation. This has been included to illustrate the importance of updating the initial narrative. Some information included here is not in the case introduction in Chapter 3. This has been done to decrease repetition.

EXAMPLE CASE FORMULATION FOR RASHEEDA: BRIEF HOLISTIC CLIENT NARRATIVE

Rasheeda is a 33-year-old cisgender multiracial woman who identifies as bisexual. She describes family, both the family she grew up with and having a family of her own, as important values for her. Currently, Rasheeda is single and actively seeking a romantic relationship. Since she was young, Rasheeda enjoyed writing, including journaling, poetry, and creative writing.

She teaches English and creative writing at a community college. She previously enjoyed her job, particularly inspiring people to include reading and creative writing in their lives, even if it was not their career. In her second year of teaching, she was recognized by the students with an award for being an inspirational teacher. She also wrote short stories and poetry, which she described as being "therapeutic." Rasheeda noted that she had a dream of publishing a collection of short stories or maybe a novel someday. **At the outset of therapy, Rasheeda spoke of these in the past tense but gradually started speaking of them in the present as current interests again.**

Drawing from her father's influence, Rasheeda enjoys humor and laughter. Some of her favorite memories are times of laughter with friends and, in particular, her family. Although her favorite television shows and movies are generally dramas, she often watches sitcoms to "wind down" after a stressful day or when feeling overwhelmed. Although her ex-husband was "too serious," having a good sense of humor is normally important in her relationships. Rasheeda reported that laughter has helped her get through many difficult times. **A few years ago, she began watching Bollywood movies and listening to Bollywood music. She first began watching Bollywood movies to learn more about and connect with her Indian heritage. Gradually, she started to enjoy the movies and music more. Now, she often goes on "Bollywood binges" on snowy days or after an overwhelming week.**

EXAMPLE CASE FORMULATION FOR RASHEEDA: BRIEF HOLISTIC CLIENT NARRATIVE (*Continued*)

Rasheeda loved living in Colorado from a young age. Her family would go for hikes in the mountains on weekends and have picnics on the trails. She does not hike often anymore, mostly due to a lack of time and friends who share her enjoyment of the mountains. Her motivation for beginning to hike again is rooted in wanting to be in good physical condition in case of meeting friends or a potential romantic partner who share this interest. She used to go to a cabin in the mountains by herself each year for a writing retreat, something she hopes to do with friends in the future.

Rasheeda is a reflective person, as evidenced in her journal writing. She tries to journal at least once a week and has experimented with different forms of journaling, often varying her approach based on her mood. Rasheeda noted that when she falls into the routine of just journaling about her day, it is less helpful. As she reflected on this in the first session, she noted that "it seems that when I fall out of the habit of journaling about emotions, I end up more depressed and on edge." Although she acknowledged that she has increasingly avoided emotions over the last few years, she does value emotions, which she learned from her father. She noted, however, that she struggled to share emotions except in close friendships or with family.

Rasheeda described herself as "spiritually curious." Her family grew up often exploring different religions. Her mother's family is Hindu, but after moving to the United States, she did not stay active in the religion. Her father was raised as a Christian but was not active as an adult. Her parents wanted to expose Rasheeda and her siblings to different religions. When Rasheeda was young, she did not enjoy this family tradition, but as she entered her teens, she began enjoying the different religious services and activities they attended. She felt especially drawn toward religious or spiritual groups that valued nature. She is beginning to consider exploring religious groups she may want to become more active in but, as of the start of therapy, had not done so.

In high school, Rasheeda went on a couple of dates but had no serious romantic relationships. In college, she began to enjoy dating and found getting to know different people in one-to-one relationships interesting. When the relationships started to get serious or physical, she often felt uncomfortable and slowed down or ended the relationship. She had one serious relationship before her marriage and has been in one serious relationship since. She recently began dating again but noted that it was not as much fun as when she was young because she is now more focused on marriage and family. She wants to enjoy dating again.

In the first session, Rasheeda was reserved emotionally but quite open in sharing details about her life. She acknowledged being nervous about therapy but also hopeful and proud of herself for having the courage to seek out therapy. Rasheeda acknowledged not knowing how therapy works and, toward the end of the first session, asked many insightful questions to get a better understanding of how best to use therapy. She appeared relieved at the end of the first session and began smiling more.

5

Concern or Problem Identification

The focus or focuses in psychotherapy typically center on identifying an aspect of life the client would like to change. While the focus may occasionally be purely exploratory or for personal growth, it most often relates to a concern or problem. Differences in therapeutic modalities emerge regarding how the concerns or problems are identified and conceptualized. Typically, this centers on diagnosis, which is often eschewed by existential–humanistic (EH) therapists. Eells's (2015) approach to case formulation is intended to be integrative and transtheoretical, rooted in principles of evidence-based practice. While Eells prioritized using a problem list and acknowledged the limitations of diagnosis, he still believes diagnosis is important, if not necessary. This is understandable. Insurance companies require a diagnosis to pay for treatment even when the diagnosis may not be necessary or beneficial for the client's treatment. It is partly due to this that graduate programs emphasize the importance of learning diagnosis, and most training sites require diagnosis. Even if one is critical of diagnosis and prefers not to diagnose, it is still important to learn to diagnose for several reasons.

First, knowing how to diagnose empowers therapists to remove and argue against prior diagnoses that may be incorrect or no longer correct. This is particularly important when working with minoritized clients who are more likely to receive more diagnoses and more severe diagnoses (Karter & Kamens, 2019). Second, if one is going to critique diagnosis, it is critical to have a strong understanding of the foundations of diagnosis. Third, even if one prefers not to diagnose, there are times when it is beneficial for clients. For example, if a client

https://doi.org/10.1037/0000464-006
Case Formulation in Existential–Humanistic Therapy, by L. Hoffman and H. P. Cleare-Hoffman

would benefit from accommodations at school or work, providing a psychological diagnosis can help the therapist argue for the accommodations on behalf of the client.

Humanistic psychology, which includes EH psychology, has led the way in developing in-depth critiques and pursuing alternatives to diagnosis (Kamens, Cosgrove, et al., 2019; Kamens, Elkins, & Robbins, 2017; Kamens et al., 2018; Kamens, Flanagan, & Robbins, 2019; Kamens, Robbins, & Flanagan, 2017, 2019a, 2019b; Robbins et al., 2017). As part of these efforts, Lucy Johnstone (2018) advocated that case formulation could be an alternative to diagnosis. Consistent with this, Goldman and Greenberg (2015) developed their approach to case formulation in emotion-focused therapy, a humanistic therapy, without reliance on diagnosis. We take a similar approach that de-emphasizes and de-centers diagnosis; however, we recognize that diagnosis is often required and occasionally beneficial and, therefore, allow for it to be included.

CONCERN OR PROBLEM IDENTIFICATION SECTIONS

The concern or problem identification section of the case formulation template in Appendix A distinguishes itself from mainstream approaches, including Eells's (2015) integrative approach, in several ways. First, "concern" is included along with "problem" in the identification of the section. Although this may appear to be parsing words, the words have an impact. The inclusion of concern intends to depathologize some reasons clients seek therapy. Next, four sections plus two optional sections are included: (a) Client's Description of the Concern or Problem, (b) Diagnosis of Systems or Contextual Issues Impacting Psychological Health, (c) Implications of the Concern or Problem, (d) Legal and Ethical Issues, (e) *ICD-10* Diagnosis or *DSM-5* Diagnosis (optional), and (f) Alternative Diagnosis (optional). Approaches to case formulation typically include a problem list. In the EH approach, this is developed using the first three sections, with each taking a slightly different focus (subjective, systemic, objective). The inclusion of the system, in particular, contrasts with mainstream and integrative approaches. For example, while Eells (2015) considered system or cultural factors, they are not as integral to the case formulation process. The diagnosis sections, which are central to most mainstream and integrative approaches, are optional in the EH approach.

The ordering of these sections is important. The client's subjective view of the problem is the starting point, consistent with humanistic and EH approaches that see the client as the primary expert on their own experience (see Goldman & Greenberg, 2015). Next, consideration is given to the systemic impact. Beginning with these sections, priority is given to the client's viewpoint and recognition that many problems clients face include how the client is impacted by their environment. From here, there is a shift to more objective perspectives and, if beneficial, diagnosis. Each of these sections is considered later. After each of the first four sections is an example of how to write the case formulation for Rasheeda, who was introduced in Chapter 3 (other case examples are also briefly described).[1] Each example case formulation demonstrates how it evolved over time with a side-by-side comparison showing the case formulation through eight sessions on the left and an updated case formulation through 30 sessions on the right. Bolded text indicates new information that emerged later in therapy, demonstrating the importance of updating the case formulation. In an actual case formulation, we recommend updating without bolding new material. We do not include an example for the diagnostic session because these are optional. The *Diagnostic and Statistical Manual of Mental Disorders* (5th ed., text rev.; *DSM-5-TR*; American Psychiatric Association, 2022) or *International Statistical Classification of Diseases and Related Health Problems* (11th ed.; *ICD-11*; World Health Organization, 2019) diagnosis also is generally thoroughly covered in most therapists' training.

Client's Description of the Concern or Problem

EH case formulation begins with the client's perspective on the concern or problem as the client is viewed as the expert on their own experience. This does not discount, however, a recognition that clients have blind spots, distortions, and self-deceptions. Existential perspectives have long recognized that individuals understand themselves, in part, through their relationships with other people (Beauvoir, 1949/2009; Sartre, 1943/2021). This section describes the client's subjective view of the issues that have brought them to therapy. As much as possible, it is good to incorporate their language, including brief quotes. For example, a client in conflict with their partner, which includes yelling and intense arguments, may describe their experience as being frustrated and irritated with their partner. As an outside observer, the therapist may view this as anger, possibly even rage. The client's choice of language, however, is important. This softer terminology may reflect self-deceptions, attempts to present well for the therapist, or fear of being labeled as angry. However, the client's choice may also be due to their experience with emotions. The language choice could be due to growing up in an environment where anger was not expressed openly or due to cultural differences. In summary, the language choice often has clinical significance.

To illustrate, Lucia grew up in Spain before moving to the United States, where she is currently a graduate student in clinical psychology. She began dating Ben, a White man from the rural United States with Northern European ancestry. In Ben's family, emotions were muted, and strong emotions, particularly anger, were discouraged and viewed as a sign of problems. When Lucia's family visited, Ben and Lucia spent several days with her family. Lucia's family had many lively debates with raised voices and animated nonverbal expressions. After one particularly lively debate, Ben excused himself to go to the bedroom.

---

[1]The clients in this chapter's case examples are fictional, inspired by common themes and interactions we have had with our clients.

Several minutes later, Lucia checked on Ben to find him with eyes red from crying. Lucia asked him what was wrong, and Ben responded, "Everyone is so angry. I didn't know your family had so much conflict. It makes me sad." Surprised, Lucia responded, saying, "What are you talking about? We are having a great time. We just like to debate and tease each other." As they talked through it, they were able to recognize that the different perceptions of the conversation were, in large part, cultural differences. Ben recognized that Lucia's family was not fighting and were not angry with each other. Ben and Lucia had differences in what they understood as anger. Similar differences have implications in psychotherapy. At times, the therapist and the client may use different labels for emotions, such as the one between Ben and Lucia. In addition, clients may bring concerns to therapy that emerge from experiencing disconnections from friends, family, or colleagues because of differences in emotional labels that result in them feeling misunderstood.

Honoring the client's language while remaining curious about it is valuable for case formulation. Instead of assuming that a client is presenting well or toning down their emotion, it is illuminating to strive to understand the client's reason for choosing the language they do.

Similarly, therapists may identify potential problems early in therapy that the client does not identify as problems. While it is valuable to mark these and remain curious about them, it is important not to assume they are an issue for the client in most instances. For example, Rami often spoke about feeling "guilty" about things. His previous therapist focused on this and told Rami it was a negative thought pattern and that he was being too hard on himself. The therapist believed this was a significant contributor to Rami's depression, even though Rami insisted that it was not. After several sessions, Rami dropped out. When he began seeing his new therapist, he explained that he was okay with his feelings of guilt. For Rami, being attuned to his feelings of guilt was connected to his commitment to character and integrity. While the guilt was not a pleasant feeling, he valued it and viewed it as connected to his happiness; his awareness and openness to his guilt helped him live in ways that made him proud of himself and happier.

Trusting the client's appraisal of their problems opens new possibilities that are often missed through universalized interpretations of behavior. In EH therapy, there is a strong preference for the idiographic over the nomothetic. Knowledge drawn from nomothetic methods can be useful at times; however, the emphasis on the uniqueness and subjectivity of each client allows therapists to understand the client in their own context.

The client's description of the problem has three subsections. First is the section Initial Client Perspective on the Concern or Problem. After this is the section Emergent Client Perspective on the Concern or Problem. It is valuable to distinguish between the initial and emergent understanding of the problems. The first section on the client's description of the concern may be finalized within the first one to eight sessions, depending on the context. While most sections of the case formulation are updated as needed, this section can be finalized as the initial presentation, and updates can be placed in the Emergent Client Perspective on the Concern or Problem section. After this, a third section is included that becomes more prominent in the case formulation section: Areas to Follow Up or Clarify. This is a place to mark or track potential issues that have not been clarified and hypotheses the therapist identifies as valuable to explore. It is important to be careful with hypotheses to ensure the therapist does not approach these with the intent or desire to confirm them. Rather, they should be held as curiosities, with the therapist focusing on trying to clarify them. These can be listed as bullet points instead of a narrative. In this section, once they are discussed and clarified or confirmed with the client, they can be moved up and integrated into the main Emergent Client Perspective on the Concern or Problem section. Except in rare instances, the therapist should not seek to clarify these by directing the session to address the issue. Rather, the therapist waits for them to emerge. At times, it may be beneficial to review these before sessions to keep them in the therapist's consciousness, making it more likely they will recognize the issue should it emerge less directly.

EXAMPLE CASE FORMULATION FOR RASHEEDA: CLIENT'S PERSPECTIVE ON THE CONCERN OR PROBLEM

Initial Client Perspective on the Concern or Problem

Rasheeda reported beginning therapy because of her sister's concern about her isolating and overall mental health. At first, Rasheeda did not confirm that she shared these concerns; however, over the first eight sessions, she gradually reported feelings of loneliness, depression, and sadness. Her primary concern was feeling disconnected from her family and former girlfriend, Spring. Rasheeda also reported concerns about her employment, particularly increasingly poor evaluations. She used to love her work but increasingly has not been engaged. Since her breakup with Spring, she "dreaded faculty meetings and meeting with students." Dreading meetings with students was particularly concerning to Rasheeda. Although she denied grief about her marriage ending, she reported feelings of guilt and shame for having married Edward, her former husband. Over the last 2 years, Rasheeda struggled with rumination patterns. Most frequently, this was about microaggressive comments at work and poorer work evaluations; however, at times, she ruminated about her relationship with Spring. The rumination patterns often interfered with her ability to sleep, contributing to her feeling chronically tired.

Emergent Client Perspective on the Concern or Problem

In early sessions, Rasheeda's focus with Spring was on feeling disconnected and wanting the relationship back. Gradually, this shifted to acknowledging the relationship was permanently over, which led her to begin grieving for her relationship with Spring. As she grieved for Spring, she reported sadness

(continues)

EXAMPLE CASE FORMULATION FOR RASHEEDA: CLIENT'S PERSPECTIVE ON THE CONCERN OR PROBLEM (*Continued*)

over not being the person she was with Spring. Gradually, Rasheeda began grieving for her father. In Session 26, Rasheeda revealed an incident of sexual assault that she experienced after her divorce. She initially reported guilt, shame, and self-blame about what happened; gradually, this shifted to anger at the person who assaulted her.

Areas to Follow Up or Clarify[2]

- Continue clarifying aspects of Rasheeda's grief about the loss of her father.

- Rasheeda is struggling with her relationship with her mother and reports not being close.

- Rasheeda's current romantic relationship is her longest, except for her marriage and her relationship with Spring. While she has been more open than in previous romantic relationships, it is still early. It will be important to monitor for the possibility of patterns emerging that were problematic in previous relationships, or that may evidence hesitancy or not being ready for a new romantic relationship.

Diagnosis of Systems or Contextual Issues Impacting Psychological Health

Western psychology has a strong preference for locating pathology in the individual, often without adequate consideration of the impact of the system. This is intimately connected to the individualistic bias in Western psychology (see Ingle, 2026). However, at times, client difficulties may be primarily related to dealing with an unhealthy work environment or family context, the impact of poverty, or issues springing from marginalization. The diagnosis of the system is particularly important when working with minoritized clients. As Fanon (1952/2008) noted, "A normal black child, having grown up with a normal family, will become abnormal at the slightest contact with the white world" (p. 122). Similarly, Jackson (2020) advocated that sometimes what is labeled as abnormal, problematic, or pathology is, instead, "*normal reactions to abnormal situations* versus their pathology" (p. 34, italics in original; see also Vallejos & Johnson, 2020). While this section is particularly important for minoritized clients, it is relevant to all clients. It is common for clients to present to therapy because of difficulties with their environment, including systems and various types of contextual influences.

---

[2]This illustration is based on possibilities to follow up or clarify at the end of Session 30.

The diagnosis of the system is intended to normalize or depathologize the client's experience and bring context to their concerns or problems. For example, Jaya, a Black woman, was referred for an assessment by her employer after several instances of conflict with her peers. The initial diagnostic assessment stated that she had mild paranoia, depression, anxiety, and anger issues. It also indicated a tendency toward blaming others and somatization. The psychologist who conducted the assessment recommended therapy and anger management classes. In her first session with Dr. M, a Latina woman, Jaya appeared hesitant. Rather than trusting the assessment and assuming that Jaya had trust issues, Dr. M commented on this. Jaya responded by asking if Dr. M had read the report, which she had. Hearing the answer, Jaya looked concerned. Dr. M responded, "I don't put a lot of stock in the assessment report. I want to hear your perspective on what happened." As Jaya began to share, Dr. M validated her and responded with concern when Jaya described some things that had happened to her. At the end of the first session, Dr. M said,

> You've been through a lot. I admire how you have attempted to stand up for yourself, even though it didn't go well. I don't think there is anything wrong with you. I disagree with the assessment report and, with your permission, am happy to share this with your employer. The emotional difficulties and difficulties with trusting others make sense and are a healthy response to an unhealthy work environment.

Jaya was relieved to hear Dr. M's response but worried about Dr. M sharing this with Jaya's employer. They agreed to consider the best approach over the next several weeks. During this time, in addition to considering Dr. M talking to Jaya's employer, they focused on how Jaya wanted to respond to the situation. As Jaya felt validated and empowered, her depression and anxiety significantly decreased. Although she was still angry, she was more accepting of her anger and sought to find ways to creatively express this through standing up for herself and using other outlets, such as getting involved in a dance class. With Jaya, correcting the diagnosis from a diagnosis of "her" problem to a diagnosis of the system resulted in significantly improved overall mental health. Dealing with an unhealthy work environment still caused stress that led to periods of emotional distress; however, she was better able to tolerate and manage this and found new ways to confront the problems at work. In addition, she separated it and "left it at the office" so that it did not impact her life outside of work as it had.

Rasheeda experienced a number of systemic and contextual issues but did not recognize them or minimized them initially. Through the course of therapy, she was able to better recognize how the various environments in which she functioned impacted her.

Implications of the Concern or Problem

In the previous sections, the client's subjective perspective and systemic problems contributing to their reasons for entering therapy were the focus. In the Implications of the Concern or Problem section, the focus is on an objective perspective. This provides a description, without judgment, of the concern or

Example Case Formulation for Rasheeda: Diagnosis of Systems or Contextual Issues Impacting Psychological Health

Through eight sessions	Through 30 sessions
Rasheeda experienced racism and sexism at work and in some other settings. The experiences of sexism intensely bothered her when she first began teaching, but she increasingly "brushed them off." More recently, sexist and inappropriate comments in course evaluations and from colleagues were causing her to feel angry, leading to patterns of rumination. Rasheeda does not feel it is safe to address these, noting that her father lost jobs and eventually had difficulty getting hired due to standing up to racism. During her divorce, Rasheeda also believed her lawyer was racist and/or sexist, but she never addressed it. On several occasions, he told her that she should "be thankful for what she got."	Rasheeda experienced racism and sexism at work and in some other settings. The experiences of sexism intensely bothered her when she first began teaching, but she increasingly "brushed them off." More recently, sexist and inappropriate comments in course evaluations and from colleagues were causing her to feel angry, leading to patterns of rumination. Rasheeda does not feel it is safe to address these, noting that her father lost jobs and eventually had difficulty getting hired due to standing up to racism. During her divorce, Rasheeda also believed her lawyer was racist and/or sexist, but she never addressed it. On several occasions, he told her that she should "be thankful for what she got."
	Rasheeda experienced a sexual assault from a colleague, though initially, she did not recognize it as an assault. This contributed to feelings of guilt and shame, which gradually shifted to primarily feelings of anger about what happened.

problem impacting the client's ability to function in various domains in their life. For example, it may describe problems at work or school or with family relationships. It is important that these remain descriptive, not evaluative, diagnostic, or speculative. For example, a description of a client with social anxiety might be the following:

> Freddie experiences social anxiety that interferes with his ability to make friends. He reports having one close friend who he does not interact with often, primarily due to anxiety when considering initiating a conversation. He does not have any other people he considers friends, and he does not interact often with acquaintances, even at work. Freddie stated that this prevents opportunities for advancement at work. He believes, "Other people at work think I am a mess and just avoid me." He added, "My boss is often frustrated with me. He has asked me several times why I don't speak up in meetings, even when it is my area of expertise."

The objective perspective has value from an EH perspective but should not overshadow the client's subjective perspective, which is the priority. When working in many treatment settings or with third-party payers, this may be required or seen as essential. This section also informs the treatment goals in the treatment planning section.

Example Case Formulation for Rasheeda: Implications of the Concern/Problem

Through eight sessions	Through 30 sessions
Rasheeda has felt "distant" from her family since her father's death, which limited the social and emotional support she receives from her family. Since her divorce and the ending of her relationship with Spring, Rasheeda has struggled in romantic relationships, rarely going on more than a couple of dates with any one person. Gradually, her performance at work deteriorated, resulting in poorer student evaluations and annual performance reviews. While it has not impacted her continued employment, Rasheeda is concerned this could affect opportunities for advancement and job security.	Rasheeda has felt "distant" from her family since her father's death, which limited the social and emotional support she receives from her family. Since her divorce and the ending of her relationship with Spring, Rasheeda has struggled in romantic relationships, rarely going on more than a couple of dates with any one person. Gradually, her performance at work deteriorated, resulting in poorer student evaluations and annual performance reviews. **The deteriorating performance evaluations occurred after the sexual assault and her break up with Spring.** While it has not impacted her continued employment, Rasheeda is concerned this could affect opportunities for advancement and job security.

Legal and Ethical Issues

Legal and ethical issues are important to consider regardless of the theoretical framework for case formulation. While these could be placed in the case formulation section, they are placed here because they are often related to why the client is entering therapy. Some aspects of legal and ethical issues will be relevant and possibly restated in the Systemic Issues subsection of the Theoretical Aspects of the Case Formulation section. In distinguishing these sections, the focus is on legal and ethical issues directly connected to why a client is entering therapy, while the Systemic Issues section considers more of the psychological dimensions and impact. For example, in this section, it may be discussed that the client is court mandated to enter therapy, including why they are court mandated and any requirements as part of the court mandate. In the Systemic Issues section, the focus is on the psychological impact of involvement in the legal system, including how this contributes to psychological distress.

This section addresses issues including, but not limited to, a history of suicidal or homicidal ideation, difficulties the client has in adequately caring for themselves or others, involvement with child protective services, or involvement in a divorce or child custody legal case. Because these influence various aspects of treatment, including why the client is entering therapy, they are important to include here.

Example Case Formulation for Rasheeda: Legal and Ethical Issues

Through eight sessions	Through 30 sessions
There are no current ethical issues. Rasheeda acknowledged brief periods in the past with mild suicidal ideation; however, she denied ever considering acting on the thoughts. She has not had any of these in over a year.	There are no current ethical issues. Rasheeda acknowledged brief periods in the past with mild suicidal ideation; however, she denied ever considering acting on the thoughts. She has not had any of these in over a year. **Rasheeda was sexually assaulted by a colleague from work. During the course of treatment, she confronted the man who assaulted her, but she has elected not to file a complaint about this at work or report it to the police.**

ICD-11 Diagnosis or *DSM-5* Diagnosis (Optional)

The *ICD* or *DSM* diagnosis is fairly straightforward overall; however, several important considerations remain from an EH perspective. If a diagnosis is required, the EH therapist will discuss this with the client, including the implications of this diagnosis. For instance, if the client is in the military or a pilot, it is possible that a diagnosis could impact their career. Often, it is encouraged to list all diagnoses for which the client meets the criteria; however, this is not necessarily required, especially if some criteria are not related to the primary focus of treatment. Given this, the therapist may discuss the possible diagnoses with the client and how they relate to what the client wants to accomplish in therapy. The therapist and client then decide together what diagnoses to include. It is essential to stress that these should be accurate diagnoses. We have heard stories of therapists who sometimes choose not to give accurate diagnoses to protect clients. While the intentions of doing this may be good, this is deceptive and unethical and contributes to distrust of insurance companies and agencies that may require the diagnosis, exacerbating systemic problems in the long run. It is important to give diagnoses honestly and with integrity.

In discussing the implications of diagnosis, I (Louis) have had a couple of clients who decided to self-pay (thus not requiring a diagnosis) or delay beginning therapy. This is understandable and emphasizes why it is important to talk with clients about diagnosis and the implications of receiving a diagnosis. Clients should be empowered to make an informed decision about receiving therapy services that require a diagnosis.

EH therapists want to consider whether the diagnosis would be beneficial for the client. For example, if a client attending college is struggling with social anxiety, the diagnosis of social anxiety may help the client receive accommodations that help them succeed until the social anxiety has been addressed sufficiently in therapy. Another example is a client who meets the criteria for being on the autism spectrum and who may benefit from a diagnosis to help them understand ways they communicate and process information differently from others. In addition, this may help them advocate for themselves according to needs that may differ from other clients. Even if one prefers not to diagnose, it is important to be able to discern when a diagnosis may benefit the client.

Rasheeda elected to self-pay for therapy, and it was not deemed that a diagnosis would be beneficial for her; therefore, a diagnosis was not given. If Rasheeda wanted to use insurance, this diagnosis requirement would have been discussed with her, and Dr. H would have discussed what diagnosis would be most appropriate. This process would include a discussion of the risks of diagnosis. When working with insurance, this may necessitate modifying the treatment approach. For example, some insurance companies are okay with an existential–integrative approach as long as it incorporates solution-focused interventions. If this was the case with Rasheeda's insurance, the treatment approach may have been modified to incorporate some of the insurance company's requirements. This would be discussed with Rasheeda before implementing the changes. At times, this may not be ideal or even beneficial for therapy—it may even be counterproductive because it may not fit with Rasheeda's goals and preferences. However, compromises can be made in which an EH approach is the foundation of therapy while regularly incorporating some solution-focused interventions required by the insurance company in sessions. As EH therapy becomes more established with the EH case formulation approach and support for the evidence-based foundations of EH therapy, we hope it will become less common for these adaptations to be necessary.

Alternative Diagnosis

Concerns raised about the *DSM* led to the development of various approaches to diagnostic alternatives (Kamens, Cosgrove, et al., 2019; Kamens, Flanagan, & Robbins, 2018, 2019; Kamens, Robbins, & Flanagan, 2017, 2019a, 2019b; Karter & Kamens, 2019; Pavlo, 2026). Humanistic psychology led the way with critiques of the *DSM-5* and in developing these alternatives. Many models could be relevant here. For example, the *Psychodynamic Diagnostic Manual* (2nd ed.; Lingiardi & McWilliams, 2017) is similar to the *DSM* but approaches diagnosis through psychoanalytic theory and research. Other models move away from the concept of diagnosis. Johnstone (2018) advocated for case formulation as an alternative to diagnosis. Therefore, the EH case formulation model developed in this book could be considered a diagnostic alternative. Johnstone and Boyle's (2018) power threat meaning framework is another alternative that fits well with the EH perspective. This model, in particular, emphasizes the social or environmental factors contributing to psychological distress. In addition to being a diagnostic alternative, it can be integrated into the Diagnosis of Systems or Contextual Issues Impacting Psychological Health section in EH case formulation.

6

Theoretical Aspects of the Case Formulation

This section contains the heart of existential–humanistic (EH) case formulation. Each section of the Theoretical Aspects of the Case Formulation includes the subsection Areas to Follow Up or Clarify. As with the Emerging Client Perspective on the Concern or Problem section in Chapter 5, Areas to Follow Up or Clarify are for tracking topics that have not been thoroughly explored or sufficiently clarified with the client and tracking hypotheses that the therapist is holding onto loosely while gathering more information or waiting for opportunities to clarify with the client. The therapist may often not pursue clarifying these but let the clarifications emerge naturally. There are exceptions. For instance, if a client broached a topic that appeared significant early in therapy but has not emerged again, the therapist may initiate revisiting it. Similarly, if the therapist has reason to believe or a strong intuition that a topic is relevant and important to explore, there may be occasion for the therapist to guide the client to explore the topic without forcing a particular relevance or meaning. If the therapist finds themself doing this routinely in a session or with a client, it is important to reflect on why this is occurring and whether it is too directive. For example, it may be due to the therapist's difficulty understanding what is happening with the client, their own insecurities about making sufficient progress, or countertransference issues.

A common error in completing this section is using theory to make interpretations or taking an expert stance. As discussed in Chapter 1, EH therapy uses a phenomenological approach that strives to understand the client apart from theory. There may be instances where interpretations from theory or research are appropriate, but they generally are limited. Hypotheses should

https://doi.org/10.1037/0000464-007
Case Formulation in Existential–Humanistic Therapy, by L. Hoffman and H. P. Cleare-Hoffman

be placed in the Areas to Follow Up or Clarify until confirmed with the client. As in the previous chapter, the Areas to Follow Up or Clarify section can be listed as bullet points to help the therapist track them more easily. As bullet points are clarified or confirmed, they can be integrated into the preceding section. Illustrations with Rasheeda include versions at Session 8 and Session 30. To illustrate the differences between versions at Session 8 and 30, new information and revised text in the 30-session version are bolded, and any area to follow up and clarify that has been addressed after Session 8 and deleted from its list and integrated elsewhere is crossed out. Because many of the different subsections are closely related, some information about Rasheeda is relevant to multiple subsections and was included as such. The illustration was deemed important to help illuminate how information is relevant to different subsections. In a real case formulation, some redundancy may be deleted or briefly noted in a particular subsection that information addressed in a different subsection is also relevant. As information is clarified, it occasionally may be determined that it is more relevant to a different section and moved there. We recommend not using special font formatting when updating a real case formulation.

For this section, it is important to keep in mind several factors related to the complexity of actual cases and applications of EH therapy. First, there are slight variations across EH approaches, including differences in labels (i.e., protections vs. defenses) and understandings of some concepts. These are not addressed in the examples to make them focused illustrations that are more pragmatic in learning how to do an EH case formulation. In addition, aspects of nuance and complexity are difficult to address while staying focused on providing a useful illustration. Given the complexity of the EH approach, it would be easier to give a comprehensive illustration in its own book. As individuals advance in understanding and applying EH theory and therapy, they are encouraged to seek ways to integrate greater complexities when appropriate. However, it is also important to recognize that a limitation of any case formulation is that not everything can or should be included, lest each case formulation become a book of its own. The illustrations provide the fundamentals of the process and structure, which we hope EH therapists will build on and adapt as necessary.

CASE FORMULATION SECTIONS

The Theoretical Aspects of the Case Formulation includes 16 subsections or areas of focus from the template in Appendix A. The first six are common across varied approaches to case formulation. The next 10 are more specific to EH therapy. For each subsection, a brief overview of the content is provided, followed by an example of how one might write the case formulation for Rasheeda.[1]

---

[1]The case of Rasheeda is fictional and inspired by common themes and interactions with our clients.

Client Strengths and Resources

Identifying client strengths and resources focuses particularly on strengths and resources beneficial for helping the client address their presenting concerns. The focus is narrower than the opening client narrative. However, there may be areas of interest or potential natural coping strategies identified in the opening narrative that are not initially included in the strengths and resources section or are included in Areas to Follow Up or Clarify. Over the course of therapy, they may be integrated into this section according to emergent information.

From an EH perspective, areas of strength and resources are grounded in an understanding of actualization and coactualization. The self-actualizing tendency is the innate growth-oriented propensity within individuals. Coactualization, according to Bland (2026), is "an emerging construct in which [self-actualization] is promoted and cultivated both by and in relationships" (p. 325). Drawing from existential philosophy, an EH understanding of coactualization is similar to Beauvoir's (1948/1976) perspective that one's freedom is bound to the freedom of others (see also Cleary, 2022). This could be expanded to include the idea that one's dignity is bound to the dignity of others. Identifying strengths can be a way of aligning with self-actualization and co-actualization tendencies.

Example Case Formulation for Rasheeda: Client Strengths and Resources

Through eight sessions	Through 30 sessions
Rasheeda is an intelligent, reflective individual who has, through much of her life, engaged in journaling and creative writing as an aid to her self-reflection. Although her relationship with her sister has been strained for the past several years, historically, her sister has been an important source of support. In recent months, they began working to restore their relationship, and it is becoming a renewed source of support. Rasheeda has a good sense of humor and has used humor as an effective coping strategy at times.	Rasheeda is an intelligent, reflective individual who has, through much of her life, engaged in journaling and creative writing as an aid to her self-reflection. Although her relationship with her sister has been strained for the past several years, historically, her sister has been an important source of support. In recent months, they began working to restore their relationship, and it is becoming a renewed source of support. Rasheeda has a good sense of humor and has used humor as an effective coping strategy at times. **Rasheeda has shown improved openness to experiencing and expressing emotions in therapy and with her sister and brothers. She also has begun reaching out to ask for support from her siblings. As part of this, Rasheeda has taken a couple of risks with vulnerability in session and with her siblings.**

(continues)

Example Case Formulation for Rasheeda: Client Strengths and Resources (*Continued*)

Through eight sessions	Through 30 sessions
Areas to Follow Up or Clarify	**Areas to Follow Up or Clarify**
• Rasheeda has been successful in her career, but it is unclear if this is currently a good resource for her.	• Rasheeda has been successful in her career, ~~but it is unclear if this is currently a good resource for her.~~ **Currently, Rasheeda does not report work as something that would be considered a strength; however, as therapy progresses, it may become one again.**
• Rasheeda reports a good childhood with a close family. It is not clear if this is still a good resource for her.	• ~~Rasheeda reports a good childhood with a close family. It is not clear if this is still a good resource for her.~~

Biological and Physical Considerations

Biological and physical considerations are common in case formulations and can include current or past health concerns or limitations, eating habits, substance use, exercise, and sleep.

Example Case Formulation for Rasheeda: Biological and Physical Considerations

Through eight sessions	Through 30 sessions
Rasheeda reports being in good health overall. She has not been exercising as frequently and has not been eating as healthy over the past 2 years, resulting in a moderate weight gain, which she is concerned about. She rarely drinks alcohol, and when she does, it is not to the point of intoxication. She uses caffeine in moderation. She reported that, in the past several years, if she has more than one cup of coffee or two cups of tea, it intensifies her anxiety, so she carefully monitors her caffeine use. Over the past several years, Rasheeda has had more sleep difficulties, primarily related to rumination patterns.	Rasheeda reports being in good health overall. She has not been exercising as frequently and has not been eating as healthy over the past 2 years, resulting in a moderate weight gain, which she is concerned about. She rarely drinks alcohol, and when she does, it **has only once been** to the point of intoxication, **which happened on an evening when she was sexually assaulted by a coworker. Since this time, she has avoided drinking with other people but has started occasionally having one or two glasses of wine by herself in the evening to "help get to sleep when ruminating."** She uses caffeine in moderation. She reported that, in the past several years, if she has more than one cup of coffee or two cups of tea, it intensifies her anxiety, so she carefully monitors her caffeine use. Over the past several years, Rasheeda has had more sleep difficulties, primarily related to rumination patterns. **As Rasheeda continued to mention a couple of general pain issues, I recommended that she get a physical, which she had not had in several years.**

Example Case Formulation for Rasheeda: Biological and Physical Considerations (*Continued*)

Through eight sessions	Through 30 sessions
	She reported that she was given a good report overall; however, her doctor suggested that she was slightly overweight since her last physical. He recommended exercise and better eating habits to lose 5 to 10 pounds.
Areas to Follow Up or Clarify	**Areas to Follow Up or Clarify**
• Rasheeda has not had a recent physical; it is not clear if the changes in her eating, drinking, exercise, and sleep have had a significant impact on her health. She reported some pain issues that have emerged, which could be related.	• ~~Rasheeda has not had a recent physical; it is not clear if the changes in her eating, drinking, exercise, and sleep have had a significant impact on her health. She reported some pain issues that have emerged, which could be related.~~

Family and Social Considerations

Family and social considerations identify important historical and current influences on the client. In addition to the typical family and social considerations, EH therapists are interested in how emotions were expressed in the client's family of origin and current family, as well as the depth of relationships. These considerations are also relevant for friendships and social relationships.

Example Case Formulation for Rasheeda: Family and Social Considerations

Through eight sessions	Through 30 sessions
Rasheeda reports growing up in a "healthy family." She had good relationships with all members of her immediate family, though she was closest to her father. Her father died when Rasheeda was in college. He had been sick, and her family called her to come home, wanting her to have a chance to say goodbye. Because they were not clear that her father might die, Rasheeda continued with an exam and did not arrive home until after her father was dead. She felt guilt and shame about this and indicated she has not been as close to her family since her father's death. She has never been close to her grandparents.	Rasheeda reports growing up in a "healthy family." She had good relationships with all members of her immediate family, though she was closest to her father. Her father died when Rasheeda was in college. He had been sick, and her family called her to come home, wanting her to have a chance to say goodbye. Because they were not clear that her father might die, Rasheeda continued with an exam and did not arrive home until after her father was dead. She felt guilt and shame about this and indicated she has not been as close to her family since her father's death. She has never been close to her grandparents.
Rasheeda reported that she could talk with her father and sister about almost anything growing up; however, her father taught her not to share emotions outside the family. Since her father's death, she described being emotionally	Rasheeda reported that she could talk with her father and sister about almost anything growing up; however, her father taught her not to share emotions outside the family. **During therapy, Rasheeda came to recognize that she**

(continues)

Example Case Formulation for Rasheeda: Family and Social Considerations (*Continued*)

Through eight sessions	Through 30 sessions
constrained except during one romantic relationship. Rasheeda does not have many close friends outside her family. Due to this, she describes limited social support.	**idealized her father, which led her to try to follow his guidance, even in situations where this was not healthy for her, such as not sharing emotions with friends.** Since her father's death, she described being emotionally constrained except during one romantic relationship. Rasheeda does not have many close friends outside her family. Due to this, she describes limited social support. **Because Rasheeda recognized that not sharing emotions was limiting her ability to develop good, supportive relationships, she has begun taking some more risks with sharing emotions.**
Rasheeda was married for several years, getting engaged not long after her father's death. She reported this was never a healthy or close relationship, and it ended quickly after she found out her husband was having an affair. She reported a limited experience of grief related to the divorce but feels guilty for marrying her husband for "the wrong reasons." After her divorce, she had a brief, intense romantic relationship with a woman named Spring. Spring ended the relationship because she was not looking for a committed relationship and felt Rasheeda was moving too fast. Rasheeda continues to feel significant sadness about the ending of this relationship. She remains in contact with Spring, who she describes as "empathetic but still firm about not being interested in a relationship."	Rasheeda was married for several years, getting engaged not long after her father's death. She reported this was never a healthy or close relationship, and it ended quickly after she found out her husband was having an affair. She reported a limited experience of grief related to the divorce but feels guilty for marrying her husband for "the wrong reasons." After her divorce, she had a brief, intense romantic relationship with a woman named Spring. Spring ended the relationship because she was not looking for a committed relationship and felt Rasheeda was moving too fast. Rasheeda continues to feel significant sadness about the ending of this relationship. She remains in contact with Spring, who she describes as "empathetic but still firm about not being interested in a relationship." **When Rasheeda found out that Spring was getting married, she became distraught and acknowledged she had retained hope that Spring would eventually change her mind and return to the relationship.**
Areas to Follow Up or Clarify	**Areas to Follow Up or Clarify**
• It would be helpful to clarify how not sharing emotions impacted her relationships with others.	• ~~It would be helpful to clarify how not sharing emotions impacted her relationships with others.~~
• It would be helpful to clarify her current relationship with her mother and brothers. She reports wanting to have a closer relationship with them.	• It would be helpful to clarify her current relationship with her mother ~~and brothers~~. She reports wanting to have a closer relationship with ~~them~~ **her**.

Example Case Formulation for Rasheeda: Family and Social Considerations (*Continued*)

Through eight sessions	Through 30 sessions
• Rasheeda shared limited information about her work relationships and other possible sources of social support.	• Rasheeda shared limited information about her work relationships and other possible sources of social support. **It may be helpful to explore how the sexual assault impacted other work relationships and subsequent romantic relationships.**

School and Employment Considerations

The school and employment consideration section explores how the client is functioning in her school or employment setting and relevant history.

Example Case Formulation for Rasheeda: School and Employment Considerations

Through eight sessions	Through 30 sessions
Rasheeda always enjoyed learning and was successful in school, including earning two master's degrees. She taught in a high school for 2 years before beginning teaching at a community college, where she was recognized for inspirational teaching. Rasheeda's student evaluations and annual reviews were strong until they started to deteriorate around the time of her divorce. She reported experiencing sexism and racism, primarily in the form of microaggressions, at work. She ruminates about these at times, which impacts her sleep. Rasheeda is critical of herself for the evaluations she has received at work, believing, "I should be able to not allow things happening in my life to impact my work."	Rasheeda always enjoyed learning and was successful in school, including earning two master's degrees. She taught in a high school for 2 years before beginning teaching at a community college, where she was recognized for inspirational teaching. Rasheeda's student evaluations and annual reviews were strong until they started to deteriorate around the time of her divorce. **Rasheeda initially was hard on herself about the deteriorated evaluations; she stated, "I should be able to not allow things happening in my life to impact my work." She has come to recognize how systemic and contextual issues have impacted these, making her more accepting of herself.** She reported experiencing sexism and racism, primarily in the form of microaggressions, at work. She ruminates about these at times, which impacts her sleep. ~~Rasheeda is critical of herself for the evaluations she has received at work, believing, "I should be able to not allow things happening in my life to impact my work."~~ **Rasheeda reported experiencing sexual assault by a work colleague. Initially, she did not perceive this as a sexual assault; however, over time, she recognized that it was an assault. Because the assault was by a fellow faculty member, it impacted her comfort at work, particularly in some faculty meetings.**

(continues)

Example Case Formulation for Rasheeda: School and Employment Considerations (*Continued*)

Through eight sessions	Through 30 sessions
Areas to Follow Up or Clarify	**Areas to Follow Up or Clarify**
• It would be helpful to explore and clarify what has changed at work that led to the lower evaluations.	• It would be helpful to explore and clarify what has changed at work that led to the lower evaluations. **It may be helpful to explore if the sexual assault impacted her performance.**
• Clarify if anything besides the divorce may have contributed to changes at her work.	• ~~Clarify if anything besides the divorce may have contributed to changes at her work.~~

Cultural Considerations

Culture is defined as "the values, beliefs, language, rituals, traditions, and other behaviors that are passed from one generation to another within any social group" and "the characteristic attitudes and behaviors of a particular group within society, such as a profession, social class, or age group" (American Psychological Association, n.d.-b). Culture is not limited to race and ethnicity; it can include sexual orientation, gender identity, religion, military, and other affiliations. Cultural issues may include cultural identity development, cultural resources, and cultural experiences. While experiences such as racism are relevant in this section, these can be addressed more specifically in the next section, Systemic Issues.

Example Case Formulation for Rasheeda: Cultural Considerations

Through eight sessions	Through 30 sessions
Rasheeda is biracial. Her mother is a first-generation immigrant from India, and her father was African American. Rasheeda heard her parents, particularly her father, talk about experiences of racism growing up and was aware of how this impacted his employment. Because of this, Rasheeda has been cautious when talking about race at school and work, particularly pertaining to her frustrations or anger, out of fear that this could lead to experiences similar to her father's.	Rasheeda is biracial. Her mother is a first-generation immigrant from India, and her father was African American. Rasheeda heard her parents, particularly her father, talk about experiences of racism growing up and was aware of how this impacted his employment. Because of this, Rasheeda has been cautious when talking about race at school and work, particularly pertaining to her frustrations or anger, out of fear that this could lead to experiences similar to her father's. **Rasheeda has recently begun watching Bollywood movies and listening to Bollywood music to learn more about her Indian heritage. She reported that her mother does not often talk to her about her Indian culture and, instead, has encouraged her to "fit in" to the United States culture.**

Example Case Formulation for Rasheeda: Cultural Considerations (*Continued*)

Through eight sessions	Through 30 sessions
Areas to Follow Up or Clarify	**Areas to Follow Up or Clarify**
• Rasheeda spoke openly about her racial and cultural background in therapy but has not spent much time on this topic. It does not appear to be avoidance or discomfort, but rather other topics taking priority; however, it is important to monitor and potentially explore if the therapist being White and/or male impacts her discussing this topic.	• Rasheeda spoke openly about her racial and cultural background in therapy but has not spent much time on this topic. It does not appear to be avoidance or discomfort, but rather other topics taking priority; however, it is important to monitor and potentially explore if the therapist, being White and/or male, impacts her discussing this topic. **It may be helpful to explore how Rasheeda's cultural identity development and understanding of her culture influenced her response to experiences of microaggressions.**
• Rasheeda appears not to be closely connected with her Indian heritage; however, it may be beneficial to clarify and explore this.	• ~~Rasheeda appears not to be closely connected with her Indian heritage; however, it may be beneficial to clarify and explore this.~~
	• **When Rasheeda spoke of relational conflict, it more often was with men. I will continue watching for markers that suggest this is a pattern, including in the therapy relationship.**

Systemic Issues

This section considers several types of systems that impact clients, including negative or positive experiences at school and work and involvement in the legal system. In the last 8 to 10 years, many therapists have experienced clients increasingly talking about how politics and world events are impacting their mental health. This is relevant to this section. An important consideration for the Systemic Issues section is experiences of racism, sexism, homophobia, and other forms of prejudice and discrimination. There is an overlap between this section and the Diagnosis of Systems or Contextual Issues Impacting Psychological Health and Legal and Ethical Issues from the Concern or Problem Identification section. This section is not intended to duplicate these sections but rather elaborates on the broader psychological impact of these issues, while the earlier sections focus on how they are part of identifying the problem. This is a critical section from multicultural, social justice, and liberatory frameworks. It further emphasizes that many clients' presenting concerns are *"normal reactions to abnormal situations* versus . . . pathology" (Jackson, 2020, p. 34, italics in original).

Example Case Formulation for Rasheeda: Systemic Issues

Through eight sessions	Through 30 sessions
The systemic issues impacting Rasheeda are primarily connected to her work environment and include instances of	The systemic issues impacting Rasheeda are primarily connected to her work environment and include instances of
	(continues)

Example Case Formulation for Rasheeda: Systemic Issues (*Continued*)

Through eight sessions	Through 30 sessions
racism and sexism. Rasheeda experienced microaggressions in the workplace that contributed to rumination patterns that are interfering with her sleep. In course evaluations over much of her career, Rasheeda experienced sexist and occasionally racist comments from students. Initially, these had a strong impact on Rasheeda, but over time, the impact diminished, partially because her evaluations were positive overall. She still becomes angry every time she reads one of the comments, but it does not last as long. More recently, these began affecting her again. The microaggressions from colleagues at her community college have also begun to impact her more, increasing the frequency of ruminations.	racism and sexism **and an incident of sexual assault**. Rasheeda experienced microaggressions in the workplace that contributed to rumination patterns that are interfering with her sleep. In course evaluations over much of her career, Rasheeda experienced sexist and occasionally racist comments from students. Initially, these had a strong impact on Rasheeda, but over time, the impact diminished, partially because her evaluations were positive overall. She still becomes angry every time she reads one of the comments, but it does not last as long. More recently, these began affecting her again. The microaggressions from colleagues at her community college have also begun to impact her more, increasing the frequency of ruminations.
	Rasheeda disclosed an incident of sexual assault perpetrated by a colleague from work. She viewed this as a bad decision on her part; however, she had pulled away from the man and said "no" several times. Over the course of therapy, Rasheeda recognized this was sexual assault and not her fault. Rasheeda decided not to file a complaint at work or a police report but, with her brother present, confronted the man who assaulted her and set firm boundaries.
Areas to Follow Up or Clarify	**Areas to Follow Up or Clarify**
• It may be helpful to clarify why the course evaluations are affecting her more.	• It may be helpful to clarify why the course evaluations are affecting her more. **It appears that the increase in ruminations about course evaluations and microaggressions occurred around the time that Rasheeda was sexually assaulted. It is not clear if this contributed to her ruminations. Some markers suggest that Rasheeda's reactions to the course evaluations and microaggressions have shifted from being primarily rooted in feeling hurt to feeling angry. I will continue to monitor this.**
• Rasheeda reported an increased interest in her Indian culture. It may be helpful to continue to explore this, including attending to whether this could be a resource for her. In addition, it may be beneficial to consider Rasheeda's cultural identity development.	• Rasheeda reported an increased interest in her Indian culture. It may be helpful to continue to explore this, including attending to whether this could be a resource for her. In addition, it may be beneficial to consider Rasheeda's cultural identity development.

Self-Awareness and Motivation

The primary source of information in this section is observation; however, this section also requires clinical judgment. It is important to be cautious and use discretion with one's clinical judgment. Several types of client behaviors or responses may indicate limitations with self-awareness:

- client difficulty engaging in reflection, including struggles when the therapist encourages them to reflect on their experience
- poor bodily awareness (i.e., the client struggles when the therapist asks where they are feeling something in their body)
- when the client is often surprised by reflections or observations about body language

As much as possible, information in this section should be descriptive; however, it still relies on some therapist judgment.

Considering protections or resistance is an important aspect of motivation. From an EH perspective, resistance, or the use of protections, is a given. Clients both want to change and resist change at the same time. Furthermore, as discussed in Chapter 1, protections and resistance are not seen as pathology and can be healthy. Everyone needs some protections. Therapists should be cautious in using interventions that may lead to taking away or lessening the effectiveness of a protection unless there is something to replace the current protection.

One aspect of this section is identifying the protections a client uses. Some of these can be consistent with or similar to what psychodynamic or psychoanalytic theory refers to as defense mechanisms. Initially, therapists may mark (or "note" or "tag" in Schneider & Krug's 2017 terminology) these and include them in Areas to Follow Up or Clarify. As these are explored with the client, they are integrated into the main section. From this section forward, it is common for sections to start with more information in the section on Areas to Follow Up or Clarify, then gradually integrate more material into the main section. Until understood from the client's perspective, even direct observations generally fall in this subsection first. The protections need not be named as protections; they can just be described. For example, Rasheeda avoids vulnerability with emotions, but this is not called "a protection" in session.

Other observations relevant to considering the client's motivation include

- the client's attendance and showing up on time,
- the client's engagement in session,
- the client's engagement in journaling or reflection outside the session,
- the client trying out new behaviors outside of therapy, and
- the depth of the client's disclosure in session.

Clinical judgment is necessary partly because the understanding or interpretation of these behaviors needs to be done in the context of the client. For example, some clients may not do well with timeliness and scheduling in all areas of their life. Therefore, frequently showing up late may not reflect their motivation but, instead, be typical behavior for them. While exploring how this pattern of lateness impacts them in their life outside of therapy may still be valuable, it may be done differently when there is no assumption of resistance.

A more abstract aspect of self-awareness is intrapersonal isolation. Yalom (1980) described intrapersonal isolation as "a process whereby one partitions off parts of oneself" (p. 353). There is an overlap between intrapersonal isolation and self-alienation—it could even be argued that these are, in essence, synonymous with each other (see the later Relationships, Isolation, and Alienation subsection of Existential Givens). Intrapersonal isolation contributes to an estrangement from oneself or aspects of oneself and provides a barrier to self-awareness. For the case formulation, EH therapists initially mark signs of self-alienation and then watch for patterns that may emerge. This can include

- emotions being disconnected from content, including possible mild dissociation when a topic emerges;
- difficulty identifying emotions or thoughts on a topic;
- not trusting oneself or one's appraisal of one's experience, which can lead to deferring to others' opinions;
- difficulty recognizing connections between topics that are likely connected or similar; and
- being surprised about an insight that is fairly evident.

In therapy, the focus is on integrating disavowed or unrecognized aspects of oneself. However, for case formulation, the emphasis is on marking these when they occur and watching for patterns or themes. As patterns or themes emerge, the therapist explores these with the client.

Example Case Formulation for Rasheeda: Self-Awareness and Motivation

Through eight sessions	Through 30 sessions
Rasheeda is a reflective individual with good general self-awareness. She has journaled much of her life and often engages in reflective behaviors. Rasheeda is aware of her hesitation in discussing certain topics and has discussed her reasons for this. An area where Rasheeda struggles with self-awareness is bodily awareness. She responded with surprise when the therapist noted some of her bodily language, such as when she was holding her breath or her shoulders were pulled up from tension. Rasheeda's initial motivation for therapy was mixed; she came because of her sister's urging and was hesitant to engage in early sessions; however, her motivation and engagement have improved. Rasheeda avoids vulnerability with her emotions and talking about her father. Over the first eight sessions, there has been some increased vulnerability, but it is gradual.	Rasheeda is a reflective individual with good general self-awareness. She has journaled much of her life and often engages in reflective behaviors. Rasheeda is aware of her hesitation in discussing certain topics has and discussed her reasons for this. ~~An area where Rasheeda struggles with self-awareness is bodily awareness. She responded with surprise when the therapist noted some of her bodily language, such as when she was holding her breath or her shoulders were pulled up from tension.~~ **Rasheeda's bodily awareness was somewhat poor at the beginning of therapy; however, it has gradually improved. At the beginning of therapy, she would be surprised at the therapist's reflections on posture changes, breathing changes, and body language, but she now often comments on noticing these changes**

Example Case Formulation for Rasheeda: Self-Awareness and Motivation (*Continued*)

Through eight sessions	Through 30 sessions
	in herself. Rasheeda's initial motivation for therapy was mixed; she came because of her sister's urging and was hesitant to engage in early sessions; however, her motivation and engagement have improved. Rasheeda avoid**ed** vulnerability with her emotions **early in therapy** and talking about her father. ~~Over the first eight sessions, there has been some increased vulnerability, but it is gradual.~~ **Her openness to experience and willingness to share emotions in session has significantly improved. Her ability to talk about her grief related to her father's death also improved, but more slowly.**
Areas to Follow Up or Clarify	**Areas to Follow Up or Clarify**
• It would be beneficial to clarify further why Rasheeda is hesitant with her emotions. Some of these have been addressed.	• It would be beneficial to clarify further why Rasheeda is hesitant with her emotions. Some of these have been addressed.

Here-and-Now

In Chapter 2, we discussed the here-and-now in the context of therapy interventions. The client's willingness to experience and make disclosures in the here-and-now is also relevant for case formulation. In part, this reflects the therapy relationship—as the relationship deepens, clients tend to be more open to working in the here-and-now. Tracking this can be a factor in assessing the relationship between client and therapist. However, it also may be due to other factors, such as the client's general avoidance of the here-and-now or cultural differences (see Underwood, 2025). The here-and-now is considered in terms of intrapersonal and interpersonal aspects. For example, a client may be open to here-and-now reflections about what they are experiencing within themselves in the moment but resistant to exploring the here-and-now with the therapy relationship. While emotion is an important aspect of the here-and-now, this is not the only consideration. The focus in this section should be on description, not interpretation of the client's openness to the here-and-now.

Example Case Formulation for Rasheeda: Here-and-Now

Through eight sessions	Through 30 sessions
From early in therapy, Rasheeda openly discussed the therapy relationship and engaged in reflection about her experience in the moment. She reported this was uncomfortable, noting that she	From early in therapy, Rasheeda openly discussed the therapy relationship and engaged in reflection about her experience in the moment. She reported this was uncomfortable, noting that she *(continues)*

Example Case Formulation for Rasheeda: Here-and-Now (*Continued*)

Through eight sessions	Through 30 sessions
was "raised to not talk about problems outside of the family." When discussing problems, she avoided experiencing or expressing emotions. When emotions related to the here-and-now came up, Rasheeda shifted topics. Similarly, when topics related to her father's death came up, she quickly shifted topics.	was "raised to not talk about problems outside of the family." When discussing problems, she avoided experiencing or expressing emotions **early on. Discussing emotions in the here-and-now gradually improved, then in Session 17, significantly changed, with Rasheeda being more open with expressing emotions in the moment after finding out that Spring was engaged, which brought a strong emotional reaction. Shortly after this, Rasheeda began showing increased openness to discussing emotions in the context of the therapy relationship.**
	~~When emotions related to the here-and-now came up, Rasheeda shifted topics. Similarly, when topics related to her father's death came up, she quickly shifted topics.~~ **A few sessions after Rasheeda started becoming more open with her emotions in the here-and-now, she began focusing on grief over her father. She reported that her feelings of guilt were primary due to her avoiding this topic. As she worked through grief about her father's death, she started changing how she approached her relationships. This was a gradual change, but she began engaging in here-and-now conversations with her siblings and, later, a close friend.**
Areas to Follow Up or Clarify	**Areas to Follow Up or Clarify**
• It would be helpful to clarify why Rasheeda avoids discussing grief related to her father's death, particularly if there is more to this than resistance to sharing strong emotions in therapy.	• ~~It would be helpful to clarify why Rasheeda avoids discussing grief related to her father's death, particularly if there is more to this than resistance to sharing strong emotions in therapy.~~
• Some discussions suggest that Rasheeda generally avoids talking about the here-and-now, particularly relevant to emotions, in most of her relationships. It would be helpful to continue to monitor this.	• ~~Some discussions suggest that Rasheeda generally avoids talking about the here-and-now, particularly relevant to emotions, in most of her relationships. It would be helpful to continue to monitor this.~~

Existential Givens

The existential givens represent universal challenges that all people encounter (Yalom, 1980); however, they require individual responses informed by culture (Hoffman, 2019b). There is no right answer on how to respond to the givens. Rather, therapists help clients decide how they are willing to live in the context of the givens. Therapists help clients find their answers rather than imposing answers on them. Various aspects of culture—particularly cultural rituals, festivals, and myths—have historically helped individuals face the givens (Cleare-Hoffman, 2019; Cleare-Hoffman et al., 2020). While many of these have lost influence over time, cultural resources are often valuable in facing the givens, and sometimes those that have lost influence can be revitalized with meaning.

As discussed in Chapter 2, EH therapists do not thrust clients into facing the givens; rather, as they inevitably emerge, the therapist is ready to help clients face them. When therapists and trainees first learn about the existential givens, it is often thought that many of these will not emerge in therapy. When teaching about the givens in several countries, this concern has emerged from students. I (Louis) used a combination of a lecture on the existential givens and an experiential exercise to help develop skills at identifying the givens. After a lecture on the givens, students were divided into groups of three and given 20 minutes to practice a therapy session. One student was in the role of the therapist, one in the role of the client, and one was an observer. They rotated so that each person was in each role for 20 minutes. The person in the role of the client could choose to play the role of one of their clients or discuss an issue they felt safe sharing in front of their peers. The observer listened and observed for the givens in session. In discussions after the exercise, most students reported surprise at how many of the givens emerged during these brief practice sessions. If they are not aware of how these may present, many therapists may not recognize the themes connected to the givens when they emerge. It is not necessary and generally not recommended to talk about these themes with clients using the language of the givens. Rather, the language is for the therapist's understanding.

Various categorizations of the existential givens exist. The most well-known is Yalom's (1980), and it is often incorrectly asserted that he developed the idea of the givens. Although a different language has been used for the givens, attempts to identify and categorize the givens can be traced to the existential philosophers before the emergence of existential psychology. We use a version of the givens that integrates Yalom (1980), Greening (1992), and Bugental (Bugental & Sterling, 1995). Greening (1992) retained and reframed Yalom's version of the givens. While he accepted the main themes, he reframed them as paradoxes, with more emphasis on the possibilities associated with them. While Yalom's labeling and discussion of the givens focused on the negative aspects (i.e., meaninglessness, death), Greening balanced this with consideration of the positive (i.e., meaning, life). Bugental and Sterling (1995), drawing from Bugental's previous work, added consideration of embodiment. We reframe

Bugental's embodiment, connecting it with emotions. As discussed later, emotions and embodiment are not synonymous but have similarities and often overlap. This categorization of the givens was previously presented in a chapter in *Existential Psychology East-West* (Hoffman, 2019c). The five givens are (a) death and finiteness; (b) freedom, responsibility, and agency; (c) relationships, isolation, and alienation; (d) emotions and embodiment; and (e) meaning. When examining the existential givens, it becomes apparent that they are intimately connected; therefore, there is significant overlap between them. Each given points to the other givens.

Death and Finiteness

Existential anthropologist Ernest Becker (1973, 1975) developed penetrating analyses of death, including the denial of death. For Becker, death is not just about the ending of life but can be understood as symbolic death, such as the loss of significance or experiencing the groundlessness of existence. As Schneider (2013) stated,

> The monumental work of such theorists as Eric Hoffer, Erich Fromm, Ernest Becker and, more recently, terror management theory shows convincingly that, whatever else may be at issue, the fear of insignificance (death or groundlessness) is a primary motive for human destructiveness—and that it is neglected at our peril. (p. 160)

Therefore, death presents itself in therapy in various ways, not just as direct or literal discussions of death. Furthermore, reminders of one's insignificance can prompt fears of physical death, and confronting one's physical death can prompt fears of insignificance.

Death and fears of insignificance have a profound impact on human beings. Becker and terror management theory (TMT) examined common responses to the fear of death and insignificance. Becker (1973) identified one response as seeking immortality projects, symbolic ways to achieve immortality. This can be pursued through various means, such as constructing a monument of oneself, making a significant impact on society or a segment of society, or writing a book. Immortality projects attempt to demonstrate one's value or significance to the world while creating symbolic immortality by establishing how the person will be remembered after their death.

TMT, inspired by Ernest Becker's writings, sought to empirically identify ways people seek to manage the terror of death. Along with research on the psychological value of meaning, TMT is one of the existential theories with the strongest empirical support. Pyszczynski and Diarra (2026) describe three ways that people try to manage the terror of death as supported by TMT:

> (1) maintain faith in a cultural worldview that imbues their lives with meaning, significance, and permanence; (2) acquire self-esteem by living up to the standards of value that are part of their cultural worldviews; and (3) maintain close interpersonal relationships that validate their meaning systems, maximize self-esteem, and provide emotional security in their own right. (p. 404)

One's cultural worldview, according to TMT, is central to managing death anxiety. TMT's mortality salience hypothesis espouses that reminders of death increase an individual's need for a cultural worldview, self-esteem, and interpersonal attachments, which support one's feeling of significance. Threats to these are met with a strong psychological reaction and often a response. Schneider (2013) noted that this can be the root of polarization, which he defined as "the elevation of one point of view to the utter exclusion of competing points of view" (p. 1).

For Becker (1975), the denial of death is the root of evil. In EH psychology, evil does not have a metaphysical or physical reality; rather, it describes destructive or harmful acts. Therefore, constructively facing one's death and significance can have a moral component.

A powerful symbol of death is not living or engaging in life, which connects with the feeling of insignificance. The idea of "the living dead," often represented in science fiction as zombies or vampires, is a powerful metaphor, and the cultural interest in zombie and vampire movies could be seen as a symbolic way of wrestling with this theme of the living dead. Yalom (1980) argued that many people avoid death by avoiding life. When clients avoid engaging in life or withdraw from life, it may be a sign of struggling with issues related to death, finiteness, and insignificance.

Although theory and research support existential views on the psychological and social impact of death and insignificance, when approaching case formulation, it is important to be aware of this scholarship without making specific assumptions or interpretations about what this means for an individual client. As death and insignificance often do not present themselves directly, EH therapists mark events and themes that may be connected to death issues. This can include, for example, signs of polarization, responses to challenges to one's worldview, and strong adherence to a group representing one's worldview. When these are present, they are marked and observed to see if patterns emerge. If these emerge frequently, they are explored with curiosity. Client disclosures about feeling ignored, alienated, unimportant, or rejected and similar themes can point toward feeling insignificant and relate to self-criticalness and the devaluation of oneself.

Issues of grief or the death of others often prompt client reflections on their own life and significance along with grief. Various life transitions, including life stages (i.e., turning 50 or 60) and endings (e.g., divorcing, leaving a job, or retiring), can prompt such reflections. When these transitions occur, the EH therapist is attentive to themes of death and insignificance emerging. Approaching the end of therapy, as a potentially powerful symbol of endings, can elicit reminders of unresolved grief or fears of one's mortality. It is important that therapists watch for these, which can present through increased emotion, particularly anxiety or sadness; more discussion about previous relationships that have ended; frequent discussion of death or topics symbolizing death; or avoidance of talking about the end of therapy. When these emerge, it is important to directly discuss the impact of ending therapy and how it may relate to the themes or symbols that are emerging. At times, this may indicate that the timeline for discontinuing therapy needs to be adjusted to allow time for addressing these emergent issues.

Themes related to death are also connected to life and the vibrancy of life. Yalom (1980) stated, "Though the physicality of death destroys us, the idea of death saves us" (p. 7). Encounters with death or mortality salience can be valuable experiences for prompting clients to evaluate their lives and consider how they want to live. EH therapists strive to recognize the possibilities and opportunities when death themes emerge.

Example Case Formulation for Rasheeda: Death and Finiteness

Through eight sessions	Through 30 sessions
Rasheeda encountered death directly with the death of her father when she was 22 years old. She has not wanted to discuss this in therapy.	Rasheeda encountered death directly with the death of her father when she was 22 years old. She has not wanted to discuss this in therapy. **Rasheeda struggled with feeling insignificant since her divorce. Because this has been explored in therapy, Rasheeda made statements indicating this is connected to various factors, including feeling alienated from her family since her father's death, an experience of sexual assault, her breakup with Spring, and withdrawing from aspects of work that were meaningful. Since discussing these in therapy, Rasheeda has begun taking steps to reengage with life and important relationships.**
Areas to Follow Up or Clarify	**Areas to Follow Up or Clarify**
• I will watch for signs that the death of Rasheeda's father may have prompted her own fears of death.	• I will watch for signs that the death of Rasheeda's father may have prompted her own fears of death. **If present, this appears less likely to have an important impact on Rasheeda, but it would be good to continue to monitor to see if it still may be good to explore with her.**
• There are signs that Rasheeda may have withdrawn from life, including decreased engagement with family and friends, and there are signs of her withdrawing from work as well. I will continue to mark further signs of this and watch for patterns.	• ~~There are signs that Rasheeda may have withdrawn from life, including decreased engagement with family and friends, and there are signs of her withdrawing from work as well. I will continue to mark further signs of this and watch for patterns.~~
• Because Rasheeda has withdrawn from people and life, she may be experiencing a loss of significance.	• ~~Because Rasheeda has withdrawn from people and life, she may be experiencing a loss of significance.~~

Example Case Formulation for Rasheeda: Death and Finiteness (*Continued*)

Through eight sessions	Through 30 sessions
• The ending of Rasheeda's marriage and her fears of running out of time to have a family with children is a painful loss for her that may indicate a loss of her feelings of significance or potential significance. I will continue watching for markers and patterns with this theme to clarify it.	• The ending of Rasheeda's marriage and her fears of running out of time to have a family with children is a painful loss for her that may indicate a loss of her feelings of significance or potential significance. ~~I will continue watching for markers and patterns with this theme to clarify it.~~ **The ending of her marriage has been worked through enough that it no longer causes distress, but Rasheeda continues to struggle with sadness about possibly running out of time for a family with children.**

Freedom, Responsibility, and Agency

Existential perspectives on freedom are complex, contrasting with how freedom is often discussed in popular culture. When considering freedom, it is important to include the relationship between political freedom (i.e., liberty) and existential freedom. Political freedom and liberty are relevant to and impact existential freedom, and existential conceptions of freedom can enhance one's understanding of political freedom or liberty. In other words, existential perspectives on freedom may deepen the understanding of how liberty could be sought. While freedom and liberty are often used interchangeably, liberty refers to being uninhibited by restrictions on one's way of life, while freedom refers to the ability to behave, act, or speak as one wants. As Gordon Lewis (1995) noted, "One cannot give an Other his freedom, only his liberty" (p. 69). Few have considered this issue as deeply or personally as Vicktor Frankl (1984):

> We who lived in concentration camps can remember the men who walked through the huts comforting others, giving away their last piece of bread. They may have been few in number, but they offer sufficient proof that everything can be taken from a man but one thing: the last of the human freedoms—to choose one's attitude in any given set of circumstances, to choose one's own way. (pp. 65–66)

This powerful quote demonstrates that while one's freedoms can be restricted, some freedoms cannot be taken away.

From existential philosophical and psychological perspectives, including EH psychology, the enhancement of personal freedom is fundamentally connected to ethics and the good life, and liberty also has value. However, it is not only political factors that constrict one's freedom; various biological, intrapersonal, social, and environmental factors also restrict one's freedom. Therefore, freedom needs to be examined in the context of the ineludibly connected themes. Because freedom is essential to ethics and the good life, it is a cornerstone of existential therapy. In the most concise definition of EH therapy offered, Rollo May (1981) stated, "The purpose of psychotherapy is to set people free" (p. 19).

Existential perspectives on freedom require consideration of several interconnected themes: (a) agency, (b) destiny or the limits of freedom, (c) the interconnectedness of freedom, and (d) the ethical dimension of freedom. We consider each of these and their relevance for case formulation. Each of these builds from each other with some overlap.

Agency. The APA Dictionary of Psychology (American Psychological Association, n.d.-a) defines agency as "the state of being active, usually in the service of a goal, or of having the power and capability to produce an effect or exert influence." From an existential perspective, agency is using or enacting one's will, which can be contrasted with being passive or passively going along with influencing factors. Such passivity avoids taking responsibility for one's life. Sartre (1943/2021) referred to denying one's freedom or pretending we are not free as *bad faith.* Van Deurzen and Kenward (2005) noted, "Being in bad faith is to opt for self-deception" (p. 14) and described it as "an active evasion of duty" (p. 14).

One of the most profound examples of avoiding freedom and responsibility is seen in Camus's (1942/1988) novel *The Stranger.* Meursault, the lead character, is living a passive life. He views and describes his life in a detached manner, including simply going along with what his girlfriend and others in his life want. Then, Meursault kills a man. Again, he describes this in a detached manner. After being arrested and put on trial, Meursault begins to reflect instead of just observing in a detached manner. He starts to consider how he is viewed and his responsibility. In doing this, he begins taking responsibility for his life. When he begins to take responsibility, agency emerges as well. The tragedy is that Meursault first begins to engage his freedom or agency when his freedom becomes restricted. This does not suggest that Meursault was innocent. Not recognizing one's responsibility does not absolve one of responsibility for their life. Instead, it could be argued that reflection and seeking self-awareness have moral implications, even a moral imperative.

In existential case formulation, attentiveness to where the client is avoiding agency and responsibility in their life is valuable. It also is important to be aware of where the client takes responsibility or takes too much responsibility. A nonjudgmental frame is maintained with this awareness. While there are exceptions, EH therapists do not assume where the client is avoiding responsibility; rather, they assist the client in considering or exploring where they may be avoiding responsibility. It is imperative to recognize that freedom can be frightening, even terrifying. This is why Fromm (1941), Yalom (1980), and May (1981) all talk about escaping from freedom. Recognizing that freedom is terrifying informs working empathetically with clients both in case formulation and therapy.

Destiny and the limits of freedom. Freedom is not absolute. Rollo May (1981) emphasized that freedom can only be understood in the context of destiny. May's understanding of destiny differs from popular understandings of this word that view destiny as preordained or predetermined. May (1981) defined destiny as "the pattern of limits and talents that constitutes the 'givens' in life" (p. 89). People encounter destiny on different levels, according to May, including cosmic (i.e., life and death), genetic (i.e., one's genetic composition), cultural (i.e., the culture that we are "thrown" into), and circumstantial (i.e., impactful events in the environment and world). These are not intended to be all-inclusive but illustrate aspects of one's existence that cannot be controlled or fully overcome. Freedom is understood in how individuals respond to these limits or their destiny. For May, even if there are many factors of life that are determined, that which is not determined is of great interest. In other words, even if individuals are largely determined, the limited degree to which one can exert freedom is of great interest and importance. EH therapists align with the agency that can be exerted and build from this.

In case formulation, it is important to attend to the destinies that clients must confront and how they respond to them. For example, one may have little or no control over the development of a health condition, such as experiencing migraines or chronic pain. However, the client has control over how they respond. As discussed with agency, it is not the EH therapist's role to throw the client into awareness of their freedom in the context of destiny. The therapist approaches these compassionately and empathetically, helping the client explore where they have freedom and where they do not have control over their life or environment.

The interconnectedness of freedom. Beauvoir (1948/1976) and, more recently, Cleary (2022) powerfully addressed the interconnectedness of freedom. Beauvoir (1948/1976) stated,

> The individual is defined only by his relationship to the world and to other individuals; he exists only by transcending himself, and his freedom can be achieved only through the freedom of others. He justifies his existence by a movement which, like freedom, springs from his heart but which leads outside of himself. (p. 156)

To diminish another's freedom inevitably diminishes one's own freedom; to support or contribute to the enhancement of the freedom of others is to affirm one's own freedom. This is echoed by many social justice writers, including James Baldwin (1962), who famously stated, "We cannot be free until they are free" (p. 10).

The interconnectedness of freedoms draws one toward its ethical dimensions. As Cleary (2022) noted, "Existential freedom entails a responsibility to others because we share the same human condition" (p. xiii). Focusing on one's freedom without considering responsibility is not truly embracing freedom. To embrace freedom is to embrace responsibility. Yet, many seek freedom without responsibility, which is harmful, even potentially pathological.

Earlier, we discussed ways people avoid freedom. The recognition of the interconnectedness of freedoms builds from this. Most clients have not thought through the complexities of freedom from a philosophical perspective, and this should not be expected of them. It is not the role of the therapist to educate them on this. However, in case formulation, EH therapists mark where clients do not recognize the clash of freedoms, including where their freedom may impinge on the freedom of others. When clients focus on their freedom without consideration of others, conflict ensues. As Emmy van Deurzen (2026) stated, "One person's freedom can become another person's oppression" (p. 442). Similarly, when one denies, restricts, or disavows one's freedom, problems almost inevitably follow. As van Deurzen (2026) stated, "Trying to control human freedom is something that always backfires" (p. 442).

Ethical dimensions of freedom. Ethics, including integrity and character, are foundational to existential philosophy and EH therapy (see Beauvoir 1948/1976; Cleary, 2022; Mendelowitz, 2008). Rollo May (1981) noted, "Freedom without compassion is demoniacal. Without compassion, freedom can be self-righteous, inhuman, self-centered, and cruel" (p. 230). Freedom is central to ethical living and living well, which, according to Frankl (1984), is key to happiness.

The ethical dimension demonstrates why social justice is always relevant to therapy. Building from the interconnectedness of freedom, one's dignity is connected to the dignity of others. Therefore, any time a client engages in behavior that negatively impacts the freedom or dignity of another, they impinge on their own freedom and dignity and likely their mental health. Therefore, when clients engage in such behavior, it should be marked to help identify patterns that can be explored with clients. While EH therapists strive to avoid imposing values on their clients, it is valuable to help clients recognize the impact of their attitudes and behaviors on others and how this also impacts themselves.

Example Case Formulation for Rasheeda: Freedom, Responsibility, and Agency

Through eight sessions	Through 30 sessions
Beginning with the death of her father, Rasheeda began withdrawing from engaging freedom and choice in many aspects of her life, including her marriage. Aside from advocating for living close to her family, she went along with Edward's decisions. Rasheeda feels as if her freedom is restricted or limited at work, including feeling unable to address microaggressions that she regularly faces.	Beginning with the death of her father, Rasheeda began withdrawing from engaging freedom and choice in many aspects of her life, including her marriage. Aside from advocating for living close to her family, she went along with Edward's decisions. Rasheeda feels as if her freedom is restricted or limited at work, including feeling unable to address microaggressions that she regularly faces. **Rasheeda has begun considering a different response to microaggressions, racism, and sexism at her work but has not enacted any of these.**
Areas to Follow Up or Clarify	**Areas to Follow Up or Clarify**
• A couple of markers have been identified suggesting that Rasheeda's awareness of her father's work experiences with racism has made it difficult for her to consider options for standing up to microaggressions and racism and sexism at work—even leading to her "feeling unable" to respond to these.	• A couple of markers have been identified suggesting that Rasheeda's awareness of her father's work experiences with racism has made it difficult for her to consider options for standing up to microaggressions and racism and sexism at work—even leading to her "feeling unable" to respond to these. **A couple of**

Example Case Formulation for Rasheeda: Freedom, Responsibility, and Agency (*Continued*)

Through eight sessions	Through 30 sessions
	markers suggest that Rasheeda is considering how her father's experiences with racism at work impacted her.
• Rasheeda briefly mentioned feeling that she is failing colleagues and students from marginalized groups at the community college where she teaches by not standing up to microaggressions. It would be helpful to explore this more.	• Rasheeda briefly mentioned feeling that she is failing colleagues and students from marginalized groups at the community college where she teaches by not standing up to microaggressions. It would be helpful to explore this more. **Markers emerged suggesting Rasheeda recognizes that her freedom and her colleagues' freedom are connected. It appears she may be experiencing some existential guilt related to this.**
• Rasheeda is avoiding making decisions in areas of her life, which contributes to her withdrawing from engagement with life.	• Rasheeda is avoiding making decisions in areas of her life, which contributes to her withdrawing from engagement with life. **This is improving but is still present.**

Relationships, Isolation, and Alienation

Humans are inherently relational beings living in an interpersonal and social context. Relationships are fundamental to one's mental health. The relational needs of specific individuals are unique. For most people, relationships are a primary source of meaning, essential to how they cope and regulate their emotions, and an important source of information contributing to self-understanding. Relationships are tied to nearly all issues clients bring to therapy. An emphasis within EH therapy is on relational depth, both in the therapy relationship and in helping clients cultivate relational depth outside of therapy. There is an inherent risk with this in terms of values and preferences. It is important that the value of relational depth is not imposed on clients.

Definitional challenges surface when examining the existential literature related to relationships; therefore, it is important to begin by clarifying important terminology, including intrapersonal isolation, interpersonal isolation, loneliness, existential isolation, existential loneliness, and alienation, including self-alienation. These terms are, as is evident, closely related, with some degree of overlap. In addition, there are different usages in the professional literature, contributing to confusion about these terms. This section is the most philosophically dense in the book; however, parsing out the differences deepens one's understanding of nuances in client experiences.

Intrapersonal isolation. Intrapersonal isolation was discussed earlier as it relates to self-awareness. Being isolated, estranged, or alienated from oneself impacts one's ability to establish a deep relationship with others. Therefore, at times, intrapersonal isolation is a contributing factor to loneliness or isolation. In the contemporary world, social media contributes to forms of intrapersonal isolation. For example, one's online presence may differ from how they interact with people in person. Thus, our different presentations or experiences of ourselves in different contexts can contribute to intrapersonal isolation. Similarly, intrapersonal isolation can emerge from one's different experiences in different contexts, which can include social media or other contexts. When an individual struggles to integrate or make sense of the different experiences of themself, it contributes to intrapersonal isolation.

Interpersonal isolation. Interpersonal isolation refers to physical separation from others. Interpersonal isolation is different from the experience of solitude. As O'Donohue (1998) noted, solitude is an important part of being with people. He clarified that it differs from loneliness, which could apply to interpersonal isolation: "Solitude is one of the most precious things in the human spirit. It is different from loneliness. When you are lonely, you become acutely conscious of your own separation. Solitude can be a homecoming to your own deepest belonging" (O'Donohue, 1998, pp. 86–87). In solitude, one connects with oneself in a way that prepares them for relationships, including deeper relationships with others. It can be a form of relational depth with oneself. Having deep, healthy relationships with others often helps one enjoy and benefit from solitude more deeply as well. To summarize, different ways of being with oneself have different consequences for mental and interpersonal health. At times, helping clients learn to cultivate and enjoy solitude facilitates successfully addressing both intrapersonal and interpersonal isolation.

As discussed with intrapersonal isolation, technology and social media can contribute to intrapersonal isolation or self-alienation. Therefore, if a person is highly active in interacting with people on social media, but this is not genuine, it can contribute to a sense of interpersonal isolation. For others, even interacting genuinely through social media, if not combined with in-person interactions, it will contribute to a sense of interpersonal isolation. However, social media may help other people feel less interpersonally isolated. Given the variations, depending on the person, it is important to be cautious with assumptions regarding a client's social media use and their experience of intrapersonal and interpersonal isolation.

In case formulation, it is important to attend to and explore how a client experiences their time apart from other people. This has implications for treatment planning as well. For instance, if a client presents with issues of isolation and loneliness and also has difficulty being alone without intense anxiety, it may be important to begin by working with the client to clarify and address intrapersonal isolation before working toward relational depth with others. Without knowing themself, they may be more prone to being influenced by or losing themselves in their relationships with others. At other times, when a client experiences intrapersonal isolation in the form of disparate experiences of themself but still has a good sense of their values and foundational aspects of who they want to be, the experience of relational depth with others will be beneficial in making sense of and integrating the disparate aspects of themself. Relationships, after all, are essential for self-understanding (Sartre, 1943/2021).

Loneliness. Loneliness is closely related to and can be caused by interpersonal isolation. However, individuals also can be lonely even in the presence of other people, including close friends and family. At times, this is existential loneliness, which is discussed shortly. At other times, it has more to do with how they are in relationships with others. For example, Jones (1982) found that people who are lonely tend to spend approximately the same amount of time interacting with other people as people who are not lonely. However, people who are lonely tend to have briefer interactions with more people, while people who are not lonely tend to spend more time with fewer people. A likely implication is that people who are not lonely have deeper conversations.

Loneliness is more straightforward in case formulation and often more familiar to many clinicians. However, a more accurate understanding of loneliness involves distinguishing it from some of the other terms discussed in this section. When clients report loneliness, exploring with the client their way of being in relationships, including what they talk about, vulnerability, disclosures, and the amount of time spent together, is valuable. The use of the here-and-now can be a resource for clarifying issues of loneliness as well. By exploring the client's feeling of loneliness or lack of loneliness in therapy, it can become possible to explore further and clarify differences in their experience of loneliness. Commonly, clients report not feeling lonely in session, but they do not understand why this is different from their relationships outside of therapy. This informs what interventions may be most useful. For example, for clients who initially feel lonely in therapy, using the here-and-now and cultivating relational depth often leads to feeling less lonely in therapy. This provides a basis for changing relationships outside of therapy. When clients do not feel lonely in therapy but do in most or all other relationships, exploring the different ways of relating in the different contacts can help inform how clients want to be in their relationships outside of therapy.

Existential isolation. Existential isolation is ontological; it belongs to one's existence as a human being. Yalom (1980) described this, stating,

> Individuals are often isolated from others and from parts of themselves, but underlying these splits is an even more basic isolation that belongs to existence—an isolation that persists despite the most gratifying engagement with other individuals and despite consummate self-knowledge and integration. Existential isolation refers to an unbridgeable gulf between oneself and any other being. It refers, too, to an isolation even more fundamental—a separation between the individual and the world. (p. 355)

Existential isolation is not something resolved or overcome, although it may be possible to briefly experience transcending it. From a case formulation perspective, the focus is on identifying and distinguishing it from interpersonal isolation, alienation, and loneliness, including existential loneliness. In addition, it is valuable to attend to how clients respond to existential isolation. For some clients, this leads to a sense of futility in trying to bridge the separation, while with other clients, it may motivate them to try to transcend this separation, even if temporarily.

Temporarily transcending existential isolation has variances. Individuals may temporarily transcend their existential isolation in a deep conversation or passionate lovemaking, feeling connected with or even joined with the other person for a transient moment. In response, clients may begin craving or becoming consumed with attaining this experience again (see the section on the Daimonic later). As the pursuit always ends in transient moments of connection at best and often becomes more elusive as one pursues it, it can intensify angst about one's existential isolation. Conversely, others, recognizing that they can never sustain the transcendent moments, become resigned to their existential isolation. Finally, some recognize that transcendence can only be temporary and learn to appreciate it and, at times, seek it while recognizing it will always be temporary. The periods of relational depth and transcendence motivate them without consuming them.

Existential loneliness. There is a lack of consensus on what constitutes existential loneliness and how to distinguish it from related or similar constructs. We propose that existential loneliness can be understood as the experience of separation due to being different (i.e., lacking shared values, experience, or identity) and/or unable to be fully understood. This is similar to the unbridgeable gulf between individuals (i.e., existential isolation) but is rooted more in the experience of being unique or different from others and, due to this, often misunderstood. Calling it "existential loneliness" distinguishes it from other forms of loneliness in that it is rooted in ontology or human existence. We are destined or condemned to be unique and different.

Mayers and colleagues (2002) developed The Existential Loneliness Questionnaire and described it as "a primary and inevitable condition of existence . . . since all humans are born into a world where perfect communication with others is impossible and only death is certain, a basic sense of loneliness emerges" (p. 1184). While it is not the clearest definition, it distinguishes it from Yalom's (1980) conception of existential isolation, particularly in connecting it with imperfections of communication. There are limitations in operationalizing existential loneliness because many of the items in the measure lack face validity as connected to existential loneliness (i.e., "I am not happy with the way I have lived my life," "There is a purpose to my life," and "I feel helpless"). Other items are not clearly distinguished from loneliness ("I feel lonely," "I feel alone").

Often, existential isolation is described in a manner that better describes existential loneliness. It is hard to fault scholars for conflating these because Yalom (1980) himself is not consistent. In his book *Existential Psychotherapy*, which is commonly referred to as the foundation for research on existential loneliness and existential isolation, Yalom uses the phrasing "existential loneliness" three times, including once when he is pointing to and referring to what he more frequently calls "existential isolation." In addition, existential isolation and existential loneliness are so closely related that it would be difficult to develop constructs that would adequately separate them. Thus, empirically, they may not warrant distinction, even if they are philosophically distinct. Still, it is important that items in scales attempting to measure these are aligned with the theoretical understanding of the constructs.

Sease and colleagues (2022) demonstrated the misunderstanding. They discussed a state versus trait existential isolation, which is fundamentally incompatible with a more philosophically sound understanding of existential isolation. Existential isolation is ontological, meaning that it is rooted in the human condition. Therefore, it is neither state nor trait. Some individuals may be more pervasively in touch with existential isolation (comparable to trait), and others may experience it more temporally (comparable to state); however, these are temporary or pervasive experiences of what is rooted in the human condition for everyone. Furthermore, they give the example of laughing at a part of a movie that no one else finds humorous or feeling misunderstood as something that results in "state levels of [existential loneliness]" (Sease et al., 2022, p. 2). This is a situation-specific occurrence and, therefore, not ontological. Our intent is not to deliberate on the misunderstanding of these constructs in the literature, which is only peripherally related to case formulation and better addressed in a different context. Rather, it is important to raise caution in how research on existential isolation and loneliness is applied in case formulation due to limitations in the conceptualization and operationalization of the measures.

The critical difference from a case formulation perspective is that existential isolation refers to an existential separation, while existential loneliness refers to an existential difference. This still may appear to be an insignificant difference, but there is value in parsing out these differences. Because existential isolation is about separation, metaphorically speaking, this is recognizing a distance between people. There can be an attempt to decrease the distance with relational depth without decreasing the difference, but there still must be the recognition that there is, in the end, a gulf that cannot be bridged. For existential loneliness, the experience is rooted in feeling different and misunderstood. This, too, is inevitable because we are condemned to be different or unique no matter how hard we try to be connected. Furthermore, if we try to resolve the difference by conforming, merging, or becoming like another person, a loss of self (i.e., intrapersonal isolation) emerges. Whereas existential isolation is about distance, existential loneliness is rooted in a lack of shared values and/or being misunderstood or, more precisely, a state of being unable to be understood. These distinctions are subtle and will often be experienced together; however, recognizing these differences can aid therapists with more accurate empathy, understanding, and reflections. Separation and difference are qualitatively distinct, even if this is hard to demonstrate quantitively.

In case formulation, EH therapists carefully observe how clients attend to their experience of inescapable difference and the loneliness accompanying it.

While some clients seek to merge with another person or group through conformity, others may seek to become seen and recognized for their uniqueness, including pursuing being more unique. Other clients may strive to accept the existential nature of loneliness—that they will never be fully understood—while concurrently trying to develop relational depth with a friend, friends, or a spouse who deeply, though imperfectly, understands them. Alternatively, they may seek to have different aspects of themselves be understood by different people.

Alienation. Van Deurzen and Kenward (2005) described alienation as "one of the most fundamental concepts of existential thinking" (p. 2). Wood (2005) depicted alienation as "a psychological or social evil, characterized by one or another type of harmful separation, disruption or fragmentation, which sunders things that belong together" (p. 21). Drawing from this definition, there are different types of alienation. Van Deurzen and Kenward identified four: "from oneself, from others, from the world, and from God" (p. 2). However, other categories of alienation are considered elsewhere, including political, economic, and cultural (Hoffman & Islam, 2026). In some segments of the literature, as Hoffman and Islam noted, self-alienation is implicit in discussions of alienation, which places the emphasis and potentially the identification of pathology on the individual. While various forms of alienation are relevant to case formulation, we focus on a limited number for illustrative purposes. We already discussed that self-alienation—separating off aspects of oneself—is largely similar to and potentially interchangeable with existential isolation. Therefore, in this section, the focus is on social influences on alienation.

Social, cultural, economic, and political factors often contribute to a sense of alienation. In discussing social influences, Rollo May (1958) noted,

> Underlying the economic, sociological, and psychological aspects of alienation can be found a profound common denominator, namely the alienation which is the ultimate consequence of four centuries of the out-working of the separation of man as subject from the objective world. This alienation has expressed itself for several centuries in Western man's passion to gain power over nature, but now shows itself in an estrangement from nature and a vague, unarticulated, and half-suppressed sense of despair of gaining any real relationship with the natural world, including one's own body. (p. 57)

Brent Robbins (2018, 2023) drew from May in talking about "anesthetic culture." Robbins (2023) stated, "Anesthetic culture is defined as a tendency of Western culture to reinforcement states of anesthetic consciousness, which is characterized by psychic numbing, detached forms of engagement, dissociation from feeling, and diminished empathy" (p. 51). While anesthetic culture is a form of self-alienation, Robbins emphasized that it is a product of the influence of Western culture. When technology, entertainment, social media, or other similar media, including addictive behaviors, are used for psychological numbing, it can result in decreased emotion and connection, which separates aspects of the self. Similarly, the focus on technique, especially in relationships, creates an emotional distance, whether through communication skills, sexual techniques, or even potential therapy techniques. The resultant self-alienation impacts relationships as well, including making it more difficult to connect at an emotional level.

Hoffman and Islam (2026) focused on alienation in multicultural contexts, drawing particularly on the work of Frantz Fanon. For Fanon (1952/2008, 1959/1965, 1963/2004), colonization and racism are pervasive influences on society that result in seeing colonized and racialized individuals as less than human. These influences fundamentally alter the way individuals subjected to colonization, racism, and other forms of marginalization experience the world, including others who share their social positions, as well as people from different cultural backgrounds and experiences. Furthermore, many forces of colonization and racism work to separate individuals from their culture. For example, Hocoy (1999) noted that assimilation contributes to marginalization through separating (i.e., alienating) individuals from their culture.

Hoffman and Islam (2026) maintained that Fanon recognized how many bicultural individuals experience various forms of alienation:

> Fanon, from his own experience and his observations, recognizes the unique challenges of bicultural individuals. These individuals can feel caught between cultures and often experience alienation from their culture of origin as well as the culture in which they are living. There are many forms of bicultural experience, ranging from refugees to individuals who have moved to a new country to bicultural/biracial individuals. While each of these experiences have their own unique aspects, each can lead to alienation. (p. 507)

This also could apply to individuals in bicultural or biracial relationships. This alienation may lead to a person having no experience of home. They are separated from their culture of origin as well as from the "new" culture. Alienation, then, can emerge from one's social and cultural experiences, which then contributes to the experience of separation, isolation, and loneliness.

Alienation can present as relevant in case formulation in various ways. First, when considering anesthetic culture, alienation may present as detachment. Exploring ways clients engage with technology and entertainment, as well as more structured or formulaic (i.e., technique-based) ways that individuals engage in the world and relationships, can illuminate detachment patterns. These may create barriers to genuine engagement with other people.

Individuals from marginalized or bicultural contexts may experience alienation from their culture and cultural sources of meaning. For example, Cleare-Hoffman (2019) discussed the Bahamian festival of Junkanoo. Historically, this festival preserved the culture of enslaved individuals from Africa who were brought to the Bahamas. Over time, this became mechanized and turned into a celebration or party separated from its historical meaning for many Bahamians. Through this process, it lost much of its cultural meaning. In the Bahamas today, there are growing efforts to reconnect Junkanoo with its cultural and historical meanings, which, Cleare-Hoffman maintained, can be a renewed source of personal and collective meaning for Bahamians. Elsewhere, Cleare-Hoffman and colleagues (2020) advocated that reconnecting or connecting for the first time with cultural myths, rituals, and festivals is a way of reclaiming meaning and deepening one's cultural identity. In this way, meaning-oriented interventions of helping clients explore ways to reconnect with these sources of meaning can be disalienating.

Example Case Formulation for Rasheeda: Relationships, Isolation, and Alienation

Through eight sessions	Through 30 sessions
Rasheeda's family is biracial, and her parents intentionally maintained some distance from her grandparents, partly due to differences in how they engage with their cultural background. Until Rasheeda's father died, her family, particularly her father and sister, were her primary sources of relational depth. After her father's death, Rasheeda described feeling alienated from her family for several years. She is beginning to resolve this with her sister but not yet the rest of her family. In Rasheeda's marriage, she described feeling disconnected from herself and her husband. While she felt connected with Spring, with whom she had an intense romantic relationship after her divorce, this was not reciprocated. In her work relationships, which constitute her primary relationships outside her family, Rasheeda described experiences of heightened existential loneliness from not fitting in and being different. Microaggressions and systemic racism and sexism have contributed to feeling separated from other people.	Rasheeda's family is biracial, and her parents intentionally maintained some distance from her grandparents, partly due to differences in how they engage with their cultural background. **Rasheeda voiced a disconnection from her cultural background, particularly her Indian culture. Recently, she began watching Bollywood movies and listening to Bollywood music to learn about and connect with her culture.** Until Rasheeda's father died, her family, particularly her father and sister, were her primary sources of relational depth. After her father's death, Rasheeda described feeling alienated from her family for several years. ~~She is beginning to resolve this with her sister but not yet the rest of her family.~~ **She began working through this with her sister before beginning therapy and, more recently, has been working through this with her brothers; she has not begun addressing her feeling of alienation from her mother yet.** In Rasheeda's marriage, she described feeling disconnected from herself and her husband. While she felt connected with Spring, with whom she had an intense romantic relationship after her divorce, this was not reciprocated. In her work relationships, which constitute her primary relationships outside her family, Rasheeda **initially described** experiences of heightened existential loneliness from not fitting in and being different. **In therapy, Rasheeda began recognizing how her family's encouragement, particularly her father's, not to share emotions or personal experiences limited her development of friendships and close relationships outside her family. Since addressing her experience of sexual assault, she has begun connecting more deeply with some of her colleagues.** Microaggressions and systemic racism and sexism have contributed to feeling separated from other people.

Example Case Formulation for Rasheeda: Relationships, Isolation, and Alienation (*Continued*)

Through eight sessions	Through 30 sessions
Areas to Follow Up or Clarify	**Areas to Follow Up or Clarify**
• Some markers suggest that Rasheeda's experience of coming from a biracial family contributed to a sense of alienation and existential loneliness.	• Some markers suggest that Rasheeda's experience of coming from a biracial family contributed to a sense of alienation and existential loneliness.[2]
	• **Rasheeda has begun working to clarify her racial identity, particularly her Indian cultural background. This is just emerging, so it will be important to continue to facilitate exploring her cultural identity and how it impacts her relationships. Whether this may be partially from a desire to connect with her mother can also be explored.**
• It should be clarified whether her family's encouragement not to share emotions or personal information with others may have contributed to a sense of interpersonal isolation, loneliness, and/or alienation.	• ~~It should be clarified whether her family's encouragement not to share emotions or personal information with others may have contributed to a sense of interpersonal isolation, loneliness, and/or alienation.~~
• It may be helpful to explore the dynamics of Rasheeda's relationship with Spring, including the possibility that she was seeking to overcome her existential isolation through their relationship.	• It may be helpful to explore the dynamics of Rasheeda's relationship with Spring, including the possibility that she was seeking to overcome her existential isolation through their relationship.
• It may be helpful to monitor and further explore the impact of Rasheeda's experiences with microaggressions.	• It may be helpful to monitor and further explore the impact of Rasheeda's experiences with microaggressions.[3]
	• **Rasheeda has begun exploring how microaggressions in the workplace have impacted her social relationships and experience of alienation. It will be important to continue monitoring this and explore how she wants to respond.**

Emotions and Embodiment

Emotions are a normal part of human experience, and all emotions, at their base, are healthy. According to Hoffman (2019c), emotions are a way of knowing, and wisdom can be found in emotions. Despite this, emotions can be, and often are, experienced in a manner that causes distress and no longer serves the

---

[2]This has been partially resolved, so it could be replaced with the next bullet point to supplement the clarification added to the case formulation.
[3]This has been partially resolved as well, so it could be replaced with the next bullet point to supplement the clarification added to the case formulation.

client well, interfering with living a full, healthy life. Resistance to the emotion or an unwillingness to listen to the emotion can initiate the shift from an emotion being constructive and a source of wisdom to being something that causes distress and related difficulties.

We include embodiment with emotions. Embodiment is broader than one's emotions, including our bodily experience or that which is embodied. Emotions and other phenomena, such as impulses, instincts, wishes, and desires, are experienced in one's body. The inclusion of embodiment points to the reality that people experience many things in and through their bodies, and it is important to attend to one's bodily experiences. Despite this, it is common for many people to be largely unaware or unattuned to their bodies because it is often not encouraged in many contemporary cultures, particularly Western cultures. When guiding clients to pay attention to their bodies in therapy, it is common for them to struggle with it.

While many or likely most approaches to therapy focus on managing or changing emotions, EH therapy takes a different approach. This has begun to change with the popularization of mindfulness, which emphasizes the recognition and nonjudgmental acceptance of emotions. The focus in EH therapy is on listening to emotions and bodily wisdom, which contributes to changing one's experience of emotions (Varisco & Hoffman, 2025). The change in emotion is often secondary to the new ways of relating to them. Curiosity is a powerful tool that aids with this. Frequently, when clients begin showing curiosity about their emotions, they experience them as less distressful.

In EH case formulation, the focus is not just on identifying the emotions but also on various aspects of emotions and how the client relates to emotions. The frequency, intensity, and client description are important to consider, as well as the client's awareness, openness to experiencing the emotion, and views on the emotion. In addition, it is good to note how long a client stays with an emotion before shifting. In noting these aspects of how a client relates to emotions, EH therapists approach them nonjudgmentally with curiosity. At times, the emotion may be overwhelming, requiring some modulation or management to be able to listen to or work with the emotion (Hoffman, 2021; Varisco & Hoffman, 2025). In other instances, the emotion may be denied, suppressed, or repressed, and the focus may be on helping the client to allow the emotion to come forth. The client's view of emotion, which is often influenced by family and culture, should be considered. For example, in some families, anger is viewed as always being a negative emotion that needs to be eradicated or is viewed as reflecting something morally wrong with the person experiencing it. How emotion is expressed and the intensity of the expression also has cultural and familial variations. Therefore, it can be valuable to obtain an emotional history of clients, such as information on how emotions were expressed and responded to in their families.

Similarly, with embodiment, it is important to attend to the client's awareness of their body and how they make sense of bodily experiences. It is common, for example, to be unaware of or dismiss bodily experiences. Helping clients attend to bodily experiences helps them begin recognizing their value and making sense of them. For example, a simple intervention such as saying, "What are your hands saying right now?" can have therapeutic benefits and provide valuable information for case formulation. The client's response will clarify their level of awareness and receptivity to bodily awareness.

Example Case Formulation for Rasheeda: Emotions and Embodiment

Through eight sessions	Through 30 sessions
Rasheeda grew up in a family that was open to the expression of most emotions within their family; however, there were strong messages against sharing emotions outside the family. Anger was an exception, at least within the family, and expressing it within the family was discouraged. Rasheeda was aware that her father's anger at work, even though justified, contributed to his difficulty maintaining jobs. The family message was not to stay with emotions too long. After her father's death, Rasheeda became restrictive with her emotions in all settings, except with Spring during their relationship. She was particularly restrictive with anger. Guilt and shame are the emotions that Rasheeda discussed most frequently, particularly as related to her father. She also talks about feeling off "off." Her description of feeling off is consistent with depression, including low energy, poor focus, difficulty sleeping, and periods of sadness and crying. She also reported grief connected to fears that she may never have children or a family. Rasheeda described anxiety and possible agitation associated with periods of rumination about experiencing microaggressions at work.	Rasheeda grew up in a family that was open to the expression of most emotions within their family; however, there were strong messages against sharing emotions outside the family. Anger was an exception, at least within the family, and expressing it within the family was discouraged. Rasheeda was aware that her father's anger at work, even though justified, contributed to his difficulty maintaining jobs. The family message was not to stay with emotions too long. After her father's death, Rasheeda became restrictive with her emotions in all settings, except with Spring during their relationship. **At the beginning of therapy,** she was particularly restrictive with anger. **Although she remains controlled with her anger, she has begun talking about it in session and using it in controlled but creative ways.** Guilt and shame **were** the emotions that Rasheeda discussed most frequently, particularly as related to her father. **Rasheeda has gained greater awareness and appreciation of these feelings, leading to them being less prominent.** She also talks about feeling "off." Her description of feeling off is consistent with depression, including low energy, poor focus, difficulty sleeping, and periods of sadness and crying. **The depression, too, has decreased.** She also reported grief connected to fears that she may never have children or a family. Rasheeda described anxiety and possible agitation associated with periods of rumination about experiencing microaggressions at work.
In session, Rasheeda is guarded with emotions, gradually expressing a little more emotion. It is difficult for her to stay with her emotions for long, and she switches topics after approximately 10 to 20 seconds.	**At the beginning of psychotherapy,** Rasheeda **was** guarded with emotions, gradually expressing a little more emotion. ~~It is difficult for her to stay with her emotions for long, and she switches topics after approximately 10 to 20 seconds.~~ **In Session 17,**
	(continues)

Example Case Formulation for Rasheeda: Emotions and Embodiment (*Continued*)

Through eight sessions	Through 30 sessions
	Rasheeda became much more open with her emotions and stayed with her emotions much longer.
Rasheeda struggles with bodily awareness, often appearing surprised or perplexed when the therapist reflected on bodily shifts or inquired about what she was experiencing. At times, she is hesitant in her response.	Rasheeda struggled with bodily awareness **early in therapy**, often appearing surprised or perplexed when the therapist reflected on bodily shifts or inquired about what she was experiencing. ~~At times, she is hesitant in her response.~~ **This has improved, with Rasheeda often identifying and voicing recognition of what is happening in her body and the significance she attaches to this.**
Areas to Follow Up or Clarify	**Areas to Follow Up or Clarify**
• I will continue tracking Rasheeda's openness to exploring her bodily awareness; initial observations suggest that she is quickly becoming more open to this.	• ~~I will continue tracking Rasheeda's openness to exploring her bodily awareness; initial observations suggest that she is quickly becoming more open to this.~~
• There are markers suggesting the client may be experiencing some guilt and/or shame about possibly not having children, her eyes often being cast down when talking about this.	• There are markers suggesting the client may be experiencing some guilt and/or shame about possibly not having children, her eyes often being cast down when talking about this.
• Thus far, there is no clear pattern of the topics she shifts to when she switches away from strong emotions. However, it will be important to track this with markers to see if patterns or themes emerge.	• Thus far, there is no clear pattern of the topics she shifts to when she switches away from strong emotions. However, it will be important to track this with markers to see if patterns or themes emerge.[4]
	• **When Rasheeda shifts from strong emotions, the topics vary, but the most common topic is discussing aspects of her job that are not stressful or involve low stress. This has not been reflected to Rasheeda yet, but it may be valuable to reflect this pattern. There are several possible reasons for this, including the fact that Rasheeda may, at times, use work as a distraction from her problems.**
	• **There have been gradual shifts in Rasheeda's openness to anger. I will continue to watch for opportunities to explore this, including shifts in how she experiences her anger.**

---

[4]This has also been partially resolved, so it could be replaced with the next bullet point to supplement the clarification added to the case formulation.

Meaning

Human beings are meaning-seeking creatures, and this meaning serves many purposes. It is associated with decreased psychological symptoms, such as depression and anxiety, and better overall mental health, well-being, and life satisfaction (Vos, 2025b; Wong, 2012). Frankl (1984), who placed meaning at the center of his therapeutic approach, saw meaning as having a role in transforming suffering and facilitating happiness. For Xuefu Wang (2019), meaning is central to truly living and engaging life:

> People have two basic concerns: One is to survive; one is to exist. The former only asks to go on living; the latter asks for meaning. The former concerns itself with how to live, the latter with why to live, the meaning of living. (p. 7)

While meaning has been established as beneficial for mental health, not all meanings are equal. Hoffman (2019c) distinguished between sustaining meaning and other forms of meaning. Vos (2025b) went further, identifying different types of meaning, including

> six types and 29 sub-types of meaning: *materialistic types of meaning* (material conditions, professional-educational success), *hedonistic types* (enjoying hedonistic/physical experiences, health and sports), *self-oriented types* (resilience/coping, self-insight, self-efficacy, self-acceptance, autonomy, creative self-expression, self-care), *social types* (social connections, belonging, conformism, altruism, giving birth and looking after young generations), *larger types* (specific purposes, personal growth, sense of one's temporality/past-present-future, justice/ethics, spirituality/religion), *existential-philosophical types* (being-alive/mortality-awareness, uniqueness, freedom/responsibility, connections, gratitude, responsibility). (p. 229)

In clarifying which types of meaning are most psychologically beneficial, Vos (2025b) continued,

> Research indicated that individuals experience better mental and physical well-being if they dominantly focused on social and larger types of meaning, whereas their mental and physical well-being was worse if they dominantly focused on materialistic, hedonistic, and self-oriented types of meaning. (p. 230)

This fits well with Frankl (1984), who emphasized that meanings that go beyond the self are more impactful.

One aspect of evaluating meaning in case formulation is attending to the different categories of meaning. However, meanings do not always present directly. Two additional strategies can help clarify. First, the therapist can attend to and explore what appears to be driving a client's decisions and behaviors. In addition, they can help the client consider if this matches their espoused values and meanings. For example, if a client asserts that their central meaning is family, but their decisions and choices seem to reflect different priorities, this is important to consider with the client. This may be a source of internal conflict, even anxiety or guilt from not living in accordance with one's values, or it may point to different values and meanings being more central, even if not recognized consciously by the client. Alternatively, it could reflect an internal values conflict.

Second, attending to client myths and myths that the client is drawn toward can help reveal their sources of meaning (Hoffman, 2019b; May, 1991). May (1991), in his book *The Cry for Myth*, explores several Western myths that have been sources of meaning for people living in the Americas, particularly the United States. According to May,

> A myth is a way of making sense in a senseless world. Myths are narrative patterns that give significance to our existence. Whether the meaning of existence is only what we put into life by our own individual fortitude, as Sartre would hold, or whether there is a meaning we need to discover, as Kierkegaard would state, the result is the same: myths are our way of finding this meaning and significance. (p. 15)

He continues to assert that myths, contrary to popular conception, are not necessarily false but cannot be proven true. According to Hoffman (2019b), myths can reflect how clients attempt to find meaning in the face of the givens of existence. Hoffman (2019b) further asserted that there is a cultural element to how one responds to these givens: "Myths represent the universality of the existential givens and the particularity of cultural responses to those givens" (p. 278). Exploring myths that clients connect with can be a way of exploring their meaning systems. In the final section of *Existential Psychology East-West* (Vol. 1; Hoffman, Yang, Kaklauskas, et al., 2019) and *Existential Psychology East-West* (Vol. 2; Hoffman, Yang, Mansilla, et al., 2019), authors from various cultures explored myths in different cultures that have served as important sources of meaning. These include songs, movies, novels, cultural festivals, and other sources and reflect how meaning can be created in the context of the givens.

In addition to exploring alignment with externally produced myths, investigation of meaning can also include considering a client's personal mythology (Feinstein & Krippner, 2009; Krippner, 1990). Krippner (1990) noted, "Myths can be cultural, subcultural, familial, or personal in nature. Mythology is a complex and sophisticated form of linguistic representation: many (but not all) myths are permeated with symbols and metaphors" (p. 137). Personal myths, then, reflect belief systems that help organize one's meaning. In case formulation, we do not necessarily identify the myths using this terminology (i.e., referring to "myths" conversationally or in the write-up); rather, the exploration of myths is the method used to clarify the meaning.

Example Case Formulation for Rasheeda: Meaning

Through eight sessions	Through 30 sessions
Family is Rasheeda's primary source of meaning; however, since her father's death, she has felt disconnected from her family and, therefore, her meaning. Rasheeda is beginning to reconnect with her sister but only in the last few months. She also found meaning in her plans to have her own family and children. Recently, she has begun	Family is Rasheeda's primary source of meaning; however, since her father's death, she has felt disconnected from her family and, therefore, her meaning. ~~Rasheeda is beginning to reconnect with her sister but only in the last few months.~~ **Rasheeda began reconnecting with her sister shortly before beginning therapy and now has**

Example Case Formulation for Rasheeda: Meaning (*Continued*)

Through eight sessions	Through 30 sessions
questioning whether this meaning is still possible for her, contributing to feelings of loss and sadness. Her career as an educator and writer has been an important source of meaning for Rasheeda. As an educator, she believed she was contributing to improving her students' lives and society. She described writing as having dual sources of meaning derived from the creative act and the possibility of having a positive impact on other people.	**begun reconnecting with her siblings. She has not made attempts at rebuilding a closer relationship with her mother.** She also found meaning in her plans to have her own family and children. Recently, she has begun questioning whether this meaning is still possible for her, contributing to feelings of loss and sadness. Her career as an educator and writer has been an important source of meaning for Rasheeda. As an educator, she believed she was contributing to improving her students' lives and society. She described writing as having dual sources of meaning derived from the creative act and the possibility of having a positive impact on other people.

Areas to Follow Up or Clarify

- I will continue exploring other potential sources of meaning, including those found through other friendships and relationships.

- Given that Rasheeda is a literature professor and a writer, it may be beneficial to explore authors and books that have affected her.

Areas to Follow Up or Clarify

- I will continue exploring other potential sources of meaning, including those found through other friendships and relationships.

- Given that Rasheeda is a literature professor and a writer, it may be beneficial to explore authors and books that have affected her.

- **Rasheeda recently began watching Bollywood movies and listening to Bollywood soundtracks. In part, these clarify her cultural identity, which may be a source of potential meaning. In addition, it could be helpful to explore if there are meanings derived from the movies and/or music that are meaningful to her.**

- **Rasheeda has begun addressing issues related to feeling disconnected from work and writing. I will continue to attend to potential changes regarding her connection with meaning that may emerge from these changes.**

Daimonic

May (1969) described the daimonic as

> any natural function which has the power to take over the whole person. Sex and eros, anger and rage, and the craving for power are examples. The daimonic can be either creative or destructive and is normally both. When this power goes awry and one element usurps control over the total personality, we have "daimon possession." (p. 123)

In itself, the daimonic is not good and not bad; however, it has the potential to be either. According to May (1969) and Stephen Diamond (1996, 2026), awareness of the daimonic is critical, tying this theme to self-awareness. When repressed, there is an increased chance that the daimonic will negatively influence or potentially "possess" a person. Instead, May and Diamond urge that the daimonic be integrated into one's awareness and self-understanding and used creatively.

In case formulation, EH therapists attend to natural functions, processes, or tendencies that have the potential to take over or strongly influence the individual. In addition, therapists attend to ways that clients use natural functions with daimonic potential, such as a strong emotion or desire, constructively. These creative responses to challenges can be important resources for the client.

Example Case Formulation for Rasheeda: Daimonic

Through eight sessions	Through 30 sessions
In Rasheeda's relationship with Spring, she developed quick, strong feelings toward her that Rasheeda described as "consuming her." Although the relationship is over, Rasheeda still frequently talks about her.	In Rasheeda's relationship with Spring, she developed quick, strong feelings toward her that Rasheeda described as "consuming her." Although the relationship is over, Rasheeda still frequently talks about her. **This intensified when Rasheeda found out that Spring was engaged; however, she was able to address this in therapy and transition into a grieving process. While Rasheeda's pain and anger from her sexual assault had always been repressed, she was able to use this to creatively confront the man who assaulted her.**
Areas to Follow Up or Clarify	**Areas to Follow Up or Clarify**
• There are markers suggesting the possibility that Rasheeda still may have strong feelings for Spring; it is important to continue tracking these.	• ~~There are markers suggesting the possibility that Rasheeda still may have strong feelings for Spring; it is important to continue tracking these.~~
• Rasheeda has been repressing anger much of her life, including patterns of microaggressions, racism, and sexism. At this time, there are minimal markers suggesting that the suppressed and avoided anger is developing in a manner that warrants concern; however, I will continue to monitor this.	• ~~Rasheeda has been repressing anger much of her life, including patterns of microaggressions, racism, and sexism. At this time, there are minimal markers suggesting that the suppressed and avoided anger is developing in a manner that warrants concern; however, I will continue to monitor this.~~

Self-Acceptance

From an EH perspective, self-acceptance entails striving to accept oneself as one is. The "as one is" is crucial because the acceptance is not accepting a distorted sense of self and includes one's limitations, struggles, and mistakes. Self-acceptance is always in process and rarely, if ever, complete. The selection of self-acceptance instead of self-esteem is also significant and, from an EH perspective, preferred (see Hoffman et al., 2013). This is preferred partly because self-acceptance can more easily incorporate failures, limitations, and the daimonic, which are often denied, suppressed, repressed, or separated in attempts to affirm or view oneself positively. In case formulation, attention is given to aspects of the self that the client can accept and not accept.

Example Case Formulation for Rasheeda: Self-Acceptance

Through eight sessions	Through 30 sessions
Rasheeda struggles with accepting her anger and her decision to not come home in time to see her father before his death. She has been critical of herself for the lower scores on her course and employment evaluations.	Rasheeda **struggled** with accepting her anger and her decision to not come home in time to see her father before his death. **In psychotherapy, she has made progress toward accepting both. Initially, Rasheeda was highly critical of herself regarding the sexual assault that she experienced. Through the course of therapy, she came to accept that it was sexual assault and not her fault, leading to her confronting the person who assaulted her.** ~~She has been critical of herself for the lower scores on her course and employment evaluations.~~ **Gradually, Rasheeda has become less critical and more accepting of herself regarding her work evaluations, particularly as she better recognized the impact of her environment and the sexual assault on her work performance.**
Areas to Follow Up or Clarify	**Areas to Follow Up or Clarify**
• Rasheeda's acceptance of difficult emotions other than anger is unclear, particularly due to her views on not sharing these outside the family.	• Rasheeda's acceptance of difficult emotions other than anger is unclear, particularly due to her views on not sharing these outside the family. **There are markers that suggest growing comfort with a range of emotions (i.e., increased expression of intense emotions in sessions), as well as markers suggesting ongoing difficulty (i.e., delaying or avoiding discussing certain emotional topics with her siblings). This will continue to be tracked.**

Client–Therapist Relationship

The client–therapist relationship is an important aspect of the healing relationship and contributes directly to positive therapeutic change (Wampold & Imel, 2015). The strength of the therapeutic relationship is important to continually monitor because it provides valuable information guiding what interventions to use. For example, a strong therapeutic relationship allows the client to move more deeply into difficult topics and spaces. If the therapeutic relationship is not strong, it may be best to slow down the process and wait to address these topics.

This section includes an additional subsection: Therapist's Perspective on the Client–Therapist Relationship. This section was the last section or subsection added to the template and was added at the recommendation of Dr. Terri Davis. This includes a point of comparison. As many clients have had few and sometimes no close relationships, the therapist and client often have a different frame of reference on the quality or depth of the relationship. When assessing the client's view, clients sometimes disclose information about this directly. At times, the therapist may inquire about client perceptions as well. However, this is often assessed through indicators of the quality of the relationship and then described in the case formulation. For example, the therapist may note the client's ability to disagree with the therapist, nonverbals suggesting trust, the client's vulnerability, and the client's ability to work intrapersonally or interpersonally with the here-and-now. The Therapist's Perspective on Client–Therapist Relationship section includes the therapist's subjective perspective on the quality of the relationship.

Example Case Formulation for Rasheeda: Client–Therapist Relationship

Through eight sessions	Through 30 sessions
In the first session, Rasheeda indicated reservations about therapy, including sharing emotions or problems outside of the family. She has been tentative with disclosures, both content and emotions. She has shown progress in gradually becoming more vulnerable, but this is slowly progressing.	In the first session, Rasheeda indicated reservations about therapy, including sharing emotions or problems outside of the family. She has been tentative with disclosures, both content and emotions. She has shown progress in gradually becoming more vulnerable, **which significantly accelerated in the session after Rasheeda found out that Spring was engaged. Since this session, she has been significantly more vulnerable and open with her emotions. This led to Rasheeda disclosing her sexual assault, which she acknowledged she did not think she would discuss in therapy.**
Areas to Follow Up or Clarify	**Areas to Follow Up or Clarify**
• It appears that Rasheeda's hesitancy is mostly related to family messages; however, it is important to continue watching for markers and patterns that suggest other contributions.	• ~~It appears that Rasheeda's hesitancy is mostly related to family messages; however, it is important to continue watching for markers and patterns that suggest other contributions.~~
• In the first session, the client reported no concerns about seeing a White male therapist; however, I will continue to monitor for the possibility of this impacting the therapeutic relationship.	• In the first session **and in one subsequent inquiry,** the client reported no concerns about seeing a White male therapist; however, I will continue to monitor for the possibility of this impacting the therapeutic

Example Case Formulation for Rasheeda: Client–Therapist Relationship (*Continued*)

Through eight sessions	Through 30 sessions
	relationship. **As of yet, no markers have been identified that suggest the likelihood of cultural factors impacting the development of a strong therapeutic alliance.**
• There are some markers suggesting the client has had conflict more frequently with males in her life. When I checked on this with the client, she did not report any discomfort or concern with me being male. I will continue to watch for markers related to this.	• There are some markers suggesting the client has had conflict more frequently with males in her life. When I checked on this with the client, she did not report any discomfort or concern with me being male. I will continue to watch for markers related to this.
Therapist's Perspective on the Client–Therapist Relationship	**Therapist's Perspective on the Client–Therapist Relationship**
• The relationship appears to be developing steadily but slowly. From the therapist role, I feel a good connection with Rasheeda, but it does not appear fully reciprocated yet.	• The relationship appears to be developing steadily. **The development was slow until the session after Rasheeda found out about Spring's engagement; since then, it has developed rapidly into a strong therapeutic relationship.** From the therapist role, I feel a good connection with Rasheeda, **which is now reciprocated.**

CONCLUSION

There were other subsections that we considered including in the case formulation that have relevance; however, we eventually decided against their inclusion. We considered a subsection on the client's sense of self. This section would be complex, particularly given different cultural and religious or spiritual understandings of the self (see Hoffman et al., 2009; Mosig, 2006). Similarly, we considered a subsection on narratives of the self; however, this can be integrated into current subsections. We noted earlier that some subsections, such as a substance abuse history, could be added to highlight them further; however, substance abuse history and problems can be integrated into current subsections as well. It is possible to adapt the template to include additional subsections based on context.

While a brief overview of all the subsections in the case formulation has been included, it is not realistic to summarize the breadth of theory and research on the different subsections. In the discussion of the different subsections, various possibilities of what could be happening with a client relevant to the theme in that section were offered. In doing this, we tried to include at least three options. However, these are not intended to represent the only options. In most situations, there are a plethora of possibilities—more than could be reasonably considered. It is a strength of an EH therapist to be able to see many possibilities for what may be occurring with a client. When the therapist sees a restricted number of possibilities, it is easier to impose reasons on a client or miss what may be occurring. Appendix B includes recommendations on further reading to go into greater depth relevant to different subsections.

The next chapter covers treatment planning, which should build on the previous sections. There should be a clear thread between the identified problems through the case formulation and the treatment plan. No surprises should emerge in the treatment plan.

7

Treatment Planning

Although many existential–humanistic (EH) stances and interventions discussed in this volume have support across a range of presenting issues, including psychological diagnoses (see Hoffman & Lac, 2025), there are challenges in determining how to line up the areas of focus with particular interventions. Many interventions, such as presence, are relevant to nearly all presenting issues, even if they need to be adapted to particular clients. In this section from the case formulation template in Appendix A, we discuss EH approaches to treatment planning, including mapping particular interventions with treatment foci. This chapter provides a brief overview of each subsection, followed by an example of how the case formulation for Rasheeda might be written.[1] As in previous chapters, information that has been added or revised after Session 8 is bolded, and any area to follow up and clarify that has been addressed after Session 8 and omitted from its list and integrated elsewhere is crossed out. When updating an actual case formulation, we recommend against using special font formatting to indicate changes.

TREATMENT PLANNING SECTIONS

Consistent with the Concern or Problem Identification and Theoretical Aspects of the Case Formulation, we developed an approach to treatment planning that combines common expectations from mainstream psychology, third-party

---

[1]The case of Rasheeda is fictional and inspired by common themes and interactions with our clients.

https://doi.org/10.1037/0000464-008
Case Formulation in Existential–Humanistic Therapy, by L. Hoffman and H. P. Cleare-Hoffman

payers, and EH approaches. The Narrative of the Client's Desired Outcome, Initial Client Goals, and Emergent Client Goals focus on an EH perspective. Because it can be beneficial for tracking progress and understanding the evolving therapy process, the initial and emergent treatment goals are separated. Treatment goals are distinct from client goals, which represent what is expected from third-party payers and treatment settings. Understandably, insurance companies and other third-party payers may not want to pay for certain types of goals or treatment foci. For example, they typically do not pay for therapy focused on personal growth, self-awareness, or prevention unless these are connected to other difficulties or diagnoses. By having a place to focus on client-specific goals and treatment goals, the EH therapist can design treatment approaches that meet the needs of the client and third-party payers or treatment contexts. At times, these may be closely aligned, while at other times, they may be quite distinct. Even when they are disparate from each other, focusing on the client goals as well as the treatment goals increases client commitment and buy-in, which improves the likelihood of successful outcomes. With self-pay clients or when third-party payers and/or treatment settings do not have specific requirements for treatment goals, the treatment goals may be left out, allowing the focus to be solely on the client goals.

The Anticipated Challenges and/or Barriers are commonly considered across treatment approaches but may be managed differently from an EH approach, as is discussed later. The next two sections are Existential–Humanistic Treatment Strategies and Interventions. EH-specific strategies and interventions, as well as possible integrative strategies, are identified in Chapter 2 of this volume. The integrative strategies from this book and Part III of *The Evidence-Based Foundations of Existential–Humanistic Therapy* (Hoffman & Lac, 2025) are examples of integrative interventions that fit more fluidly and naturally with EH approaches; however, there are a plethora of other intervention strategies that can be integrated beyond the ones identified, including solution-focused approaches, such as cognitive behavior treatment strategies, when appropriate. Identifying EH and integrative interventions provides a structure for approaching and documenting existential–integrative psychotherapy (see Krug, 2019; Schneider, 2007, 2019a).

The final two sections are focused on providing evidence for the treatment approach. First, there is a section for treatment progress. When there is a requirement to use specific outcomes or treatment progress measures, these can be summarized here. However, the progress from EH therapy often includes forms of growth or progress not easily identified by these measures. For example, if a client feels more empowered, which leads to them standing up for themselves more and setting boundaries, it is typically not going to be identified in common outcome measures. These changes can be documented here. The final section of the Treatment Planning is Support for Treatment Approaches, Stances, and/or Techniques. This is addressed in Chapter 8.

In this chapter, an overview of each section is provided. Following this, we provide an example of how to complete each section using the case of Rasheeda.

Narrative of the Client's Desired Outcome

The treatment plan begins with a narrative of what the client would like their life to be like after therapy. Beginning with a narrative is intended to help the client and therapist create a picture of the client's view of the good life, which typically is done over time. It is more flexible and broader than focusing solely on client or treatment goals. This deepens the client and treatment goals as well. The section on Areas to Follow Up or Clarify is included because many clients are still working to figure out their vision of the good life early in sessions. There may be possibilities that can be marked for future exploration and clarification as well.

Example Case Formulation for Rasheeda: Narrative of the Client's Desired Outcome

Through eight sessions	Through 30 sessions
At the outset of therapy, Rasheeda struggled to identify what she would like life to be like after therapy. She wants to have a family of her own with children. She also wants to "not feel so alone" and "enjoy life again." However, it was difficult for her to envision what this life would look like. Rasheeda discussed wanting to be happier at work again.	**Over the course of therapy, Rasheeda gradually clarified how she would like her life to be after finishing therapy.** She want**ed** to have a family of her own with children **at the beginning of therapy but struggled in describing this. For a while, each time she envisioned this, it was with Spring. As she grieved this relationship, it was easier for her to envision other possibilities. She wants a monogamous relationship but is open to it being with a woman or man—she stated, "I just want it to be rooted in love with someone who supports and accepts me." She would like at least one biological child of her own but is open to alternative means of getting pregnant. She wants to have two or three children in total. She wants her desired future family to be engaged in friendships outside of their immediate family.**
	Rasheeda wants to be closer to her mother, sister, and brothers, but she has accepted that she does not believe she will ever have the relationship with her mother she would like. While she still hopes for a better relationship, she wants to accept her mother's limitations and the limitations in their relationship. Her relationship with her siblings has improved, and she hopes this will continue. She wants them to be an active part of her life with her family, and she wants to be close to her siblings' families as well.

(continues)

Example Case Formulation for Rasheeda: Narrative of the Client's Desired Outcome (*Continued*)

Through eight sessions	Through 30 sessions
	At the outset of therapy, Rasheeda said she wanted to "not feel so alone" and "enjoy life again." However, it was difficult for her to envision what that would look like. **This gradually has been clarified. She wants more friendships outside of her family, but she struggles to know what that would look like because she has never had many close friendships. She would like better relationships with her colleagues at work, too.**
Areas to Follow Up or Clarify	**Areas to Follow Up or Clarify**
• Rasheeda has not expressed direct interest in wanting a better relationship with her brothers and mother, but there are markers suggesting she desires closer relationships with them.	• ~~Rasheeda has not expressed direct interest in wanting a better relationship with her brothers and mother, but there are markers suggesting she desires closer relationships with them.~~
• I will continue to help Rasheeda clarify her desire to have a spouse and children. Her description of this and reasons for wanting it have been vague.	• ~~I will continue to help Rasheeda clarify her desire to have a spouse and children. Her description of this and reasons for wanting it have been vague.~~
• Rasheeda referred to her love of writing several times; however, it was mostly in the past tense. There is some indication that she would like to write and publish, but she has spoken of these mostly in the past tense. I will continue to monitor this for changes.	• Rasheeda referred to her love of writing several times; however, it was mostly in the past tense **initially. Rasheeda has begun spending more time writing again and enjoying it, but she is not sure where this will lead. There have been some markers, such as briefly considering attending writing conferences and retreats in the future.**
	• **I will continue to attend to and help Rasheeda explore what close relationships outside of her family may look like for her.**

Initial Client Goals

The initial client goals are clarified early in therapy with the client. EH therapists often eschew goals as too stagnant and limiting in contrast with the fluid nature of EH therapy and the recognition that the outcomes clients desire typically change over the course of treatment. Yet, there is some evidence that goals are beneficial and can be adapted to different treatment approaches (see Cooper & Law, 2018). It is important that these are framed and worded in a manner that reflects the client's perspective. Often, therapists assist clients in framing goals in realistic terms. For example, Rasheeda's primary goal is to have a family. This is not something that therapy can directly accomplish due to many variables that fall outside of the scope of therapy. However, it is possible to work on things that can increase the probability. In the narrative of the client's desired outcome, aspirational visions can be included, at least within limits. In the following example, Dr. H helped Rasheeda clarify what goals could be realistically addressed in therapy to increase the possibility of her having a family.

Treatment goals should be objectively measurable. With client goals, this is often good; however, some client goals may be more subjective. As Arthur Bohart stated in the Foreword to Greening's (2017) book of poetry, "For me, I would prefer a world where some insights are best conveyed through poetry, and where some experiences can only be captured in words and not numbers, although I am not opposed to numbers" (p. viii). Therefore, it is not required to conform client goals to something objectively measurable. The initial treatment goals do not need to be updated or removed when accomplished; however, notes can be added to them. In the example, notes added after the initial goals were established are bolded.

EXAMPLE CASE FORMULATION FOR RASHEEDA: INITIAL CLIENT GOALS

- Identify and clarify factors within herself that may be barriers to her finding a spouse and having a family.

  - **Rasheeda feels she has accomplished this goal.**

- Improve social support, including developing new friendships and closer relationships.

- Improve employment satisfaction.

  - **Rasheeda has clarified this to include being able to stand up for herself, being more engaged with the courses she is teaching, and developing closer relationships with some of her colleagues.**

- Increase her happiness and life satisfaction.

Emergent Client Goals

The emergent client goals do not need to replace the initial goals. These are separated to help track the evolution of goals. Emergent goals can be updated or changed as needed. It is helpful to note when the goal was added. The initial goals do not need to be restated here.

EXAMPLE CASE FORMULATION FOR RASHEEDA: EMERGENT CLIENT GOALS

- Clarify what Rasheeda wants in a romantic partner or spouse. (Added Week 10)
- Decrease feelings of guilt and shame. (Added Week 18)
- Improve comfort with being vulnerable and sharing emotions with friends. (Added Week 22)
- Develop closer relationships with siblings and mother. (Added Week 27)

Treatment Goals (Optional)

As discussed, the treatment goals are included to meet the requirements of the practice setting or third-party payers. These often are divided into short-term and long-term goals. We do not provide examples here because treatment goals are optional for EH treatment planning, and there are plenty of resources for developing these treatment goals, such as *The Complete Adult Psychotherapy Treatment Planner* (6th ed.; Jongsma et al., 2021) and other books in the Wiley series.

Anticipated Challenges and/or Barriers

This section identifies potential challenges to treatment, which inform ways to prevent or address them. There are many potential challenges, including a lack of resources, difficulty attending sessions regularly, physical health challenges, and environmental or systemic challenges. At times, resistance (i.e., protections) may also be a barrier. EH perspectives, as discussed in Chapter 2, often reframe protections or resistance in a more positive light. In addition, EH approaches may help clients use these more intentionally, often decreasing the reliance on and the frequency with which they are used.

Example Case Formulation for Rasheeda: Anticipated Challenges and/or Barriers

Through eight sessions	Through 30 sessions
Rasheeda is uncomfortable discussing personal problems or strong emotions outside her immediate family. This may provide a barrier to developing a good therapeutic relationship. Thus far, the therapy relationship is slowly progressing. Currently, Rasheeda has a limited social support system. Although she is renewing her relationship with her	Rasheeda is uncomfortable discussing personal problems or strong emotions outside her immediate family; **however, she has shown improvement with this, particularly in therapy. Despite her discomfort discussing personal problems or strong emotions, she has developed a good therapeutic relationship.** Rasheeda **has begun**

Example Case Formulation for Rasheeda: Anticipated Challenges and/or Barriers (*Continued*)

Through eight sessions	Through 30 sessions
sister, this began recently, and it is still not as strong as before her father's death. She continues to experience microaggressions as well as systemic racism and sexism at her place of employment, which contributes to stress and rumination patterns.	**expanding** her social support system, **but her support system is still** limited. ~~Although she is renewing her relationship with her sister, this began recently, and it is still not as strong as before her father's death.~~ She continues to experience microaggressions as well as systemic racism and sexism at her place of employment, which contributes to stress and rumination patterns.

Areas to Follow Up or Clarify

- Rasheeda has not identified and discussed close colleagues or allies at her work; however, this does not mean that she does not have these. I will watch for an opportunity to clarify this with Rasheeda.

Areas to Follow Up or Clarify

- ~~Rasheeda has not identified and discussed close colleagues or allies at her work; however, this does not mean that she does not have these. I will watch for an opportunity to clarify this with Rasheeda.~~

- **The colleague who sexually assaulted Rasheeda continues to work at the same community college. While she has set firm boundaries with him, including telling him to take the lead and avoid contact with her when possible, there are still work events and duties they are both required or expected to attend. This contributes to feelings of not being safe at work.**

Existential–Humanistic Treatment Strategies and Interventions

The EH treatment strategies are primarily those identified in Chapter 2 of this volume. These interventions were identified from research and several influential overviews of EH therapy; however, other interventions may not be included here or labeled differently in other texts. While it is acceptable to use other interventions or labels for interventions, the interventions listed in this section should be EH-specific. If treatment goals are listed earlier in the case formulation, as in Rasheeda's example, it can be useful to connect each intervention to one or more of those goals and modify the interventions or add new ones when new goals emerge in later sessions. Mapping interventions to specific goals is especially important when the therapist seeks to establish an evidence base for their chosen strategies, which is covered in Chapter 8. Interventions added or clarified after the initial eight sessions are bolded.

EXAMPLE CASE FORMULATION FOR RASHEEDA: EXISTENTIAL–HUMANISTIC TREATMENT STRATEGIES AND INTERVENTIONS

- Presence will be used to strengthen the therapeutic relationship, cultivate deeper awareness, and increase relational depth.

- **Self-disclosure was effective in early sessions to help develop a deeper therapy relationship and model self-disclosure to the client.** Brief self-disclosures will **continue to** be used to model emotional expression and emotion management and facilitate relational depth.

- Vivification of protections will be used to increase awareness of how protections are impacting Rasheeda's relationships with other people.

- Facilitating self-awareness will be used to help Rasheeda develop insight into relational patterns, including those that may be causing barriers to satisfying relationships. Facilitating self-awareness will also be used to help Rasheeda clarify values and what she is looking for in a romantic partner.

- Here-and-now interventions will provide a foundation for increasing self-awareness in relationships and deepening emotional awareness.

- The therapist's use of genuineness will be important for developing relational depth in the therapy relationship and facilitating the development of more genuine relationships outside of therapy.

- Acceptance, genuineness, here-and-now explorations, and the facilitation of self-awareness will be used to address feelings of guilt and shame.

- Meaning-centered interventions will be used to address dissatisfaction and disconnection with important aspects of Rasheeda's life and promote general psychological well-being.

- **The facilitation of emotional processing, acceptance, and empathy will be used for grieving Rasheeda's father's death and addressing emotions related to her sexual assault.**

Integrative Strategies

All treatments tend to be more effective when they are less rigid and open to integrating other strategies as needed or beneficial to the client (Norcross & Wampold, 2019). Some interventions, such as mindfulness, expressive arts interventions, and experiential techniques, are regularly and rather fluidly integrated as they fit more readily with the foundations of EH therapy. Other interventions, including solution-focused and trauma-informed interventions and eye movement desensitization and reprocessing, may be used when beneficial to the client. Integrating some of these interventions may even be required when working with third-party payers. Even when not required, EH therapists should consider them when they fit the client's goals and needs.

With Rasheeda, there were no requirements to use integrative strategies; however, some were included as they were identified as beneficial for Rasheeda. Interventions added or clarified after the initial eight sessions are bolded.

EXAMPLE CASE FORMULATION FOR RASHEEDA: INTEGRATIVE STRATEGIES

- Mindfulness strategies will be used to facilitate greater bodily and emotional awareness and promote acceptance of Rasheeda's emotions, **particularly guilt and shame**.

- Expressive arts and journaling interventions will be used to facilitate self-awareness and emotional expression.

- **Breathing techniques for emotional regulation will be used to help manage emotions related to Rasheeda's experience of sexual assault. These will also be used to promote better sleep.**

Treatment Progress

The treatment progress section includes a mixture of the client's subjective appraisals of improvement, the therapist's observations of change, and summaries of outcome measures used (if applicable). This helps demonstrate what has been effective in treatment. It can also be used to track and demonstrate what has not been effective. For example, if working with a client who has a negative reaction to cognitive behavior or solution-focused interventions, this can be noted here. In contexts where these interventions are strongly encouraged or required, this can provide information clarifying why "preferred treatment approaches" are no longer being incorporated.

Example Case Formulation for Rasheeda: Treatment Progress

Through eight sessions	Through 30 sessions
Rasheeda reported a decrease in overall distress and some decrease in feelings of isolation and loneliness, largely due to the therapy relationship. She reported feeling better after sessions in which there was some emotional disclosure. There has been some improvement in self-awareness, including recognizing how interpersonal patterns have discouraged closer relationships.	Rasheeda reports a **significant** decrease in distress and feelings of isolation, **which she attributes to the therapy relationship and connecting more deeply with her sister and brothers again. Rasheeda has taken more risks with being vulnerable, which contributed to feeling more connected with others. Although she still has periods of feeling lonely and isolated, these are less frequent and less severe.**

(continues)

Example Case Formulation for Rasheeda: Treatment Progress (*Continued*)

Through eight sessions	Through 30 sessions
	She is increasingly aware that she feels better after sessions when she expresses and processes emotions. Her self-awareness **has continued to improve,** including recognizing how some interpersonal patterns have discouraged closer relationships.
	Rasheeda made progress in accepting her relationship with Spring is over and grieving for this. She also progressed with grieving the death of her father, which contributed to decreased guilt and shame. As these were resolved, she has more easily explored and envisioned what she would like her life to be like after therapy. She also feels more prepared to begin dating again.
	Rasheeda recently disclosed a trauma—having been sexually assaulted. Since then, she has made significant progress in processing her emotions, decreasing their frequency and intensity. She no longer blames herself for what happened. Rasheeda has felt more empowered, which resulted in her confronting the man who sexually assaulted her and setting firm boundaries with him. She also feels slightly more empowered in facing microaggressions and systemic racism and sexism at work. Rasheeda has not addressed these at work yet but is considering how she would like to approach this.
	Rasheeda reports that she is now happy with her life most of the time, but she still has concerns she wants to address in therapy. She is more hopeful and confident that she will successfully address them.

CONCLUSION

EH treatment planning can be integrated into mainstream approaches by incorporating client goals and EH interventions alongside other goals and treatment strategies. In addition, an EH framework can integrate various approaches to evaluating the effectiveness of treatment, including outcome measures, process measures, the client's subjective appraisals, and the therapist's observations. Moreover, a strategy whereby EH therapists can demonstrate the research foundations of their treatment strategies can be incorporated, which is discussed in Chapter 8.

8

Support for Treatment Approaches, Stances, and/or Techniques

While it may not always be necessary to demonstrate that the therapist is practicing consistent with evidence-based practice in psychology (EBPP) with every client or in all contexts, all existential–humanistic (EH) therapists should know how to do so. Furthermore, it is the responsibility of all therapists to regularly critically assess the effectiveness of their approach to therapy in the context of theory, research, practice-based evidence, and other sources of information as part of one's care and commitment to one's clients.

The companion book to this volume, *The Evidence-Based Foundations of Existential–Humanistic Therapy* (Hoffman & Lac, 2025), reviews the evidence on EH interventions and how they can be adapted for cultural differences. Therefore, we do not review the evidence here but briefly provide an overview of the framework for supporting that one is practicing consistent with EBPP with individual clients.

EVIDENCE-BASED PSYCHOLOGICAL PRACTICE AND EXISTENTIAL–HUMANISTIC THERAPY

The seminal article in the *American Psychologist* on EBPP sets forth the criteria for practicing consistent with EBPP standards (American Psychological Association, Presidential Task Force on Evidence-Based Practice, 2006). There are three pillars to EBPP: (a) best available research evidence; (b) clinical experience; and (c) client characteristics, culture, and preference. Each of these needs to

https://doi.org/10.1037/0000464-009
Case Formulation in Existential–Humanistic Therapy, by L. Hoffman and H. P. Cleare-Hoffman

157

be considered when assessing one's practice; however, the emphasis too often falls solely on research. These three facets are aspects of treatment that the therapist must address, not criteria to establish any modality as an EBPP. In fact, it is a misunderstanding of EBPP to refer to any modality as an evidence-based practice. Hoffman (2024) stated that EBPP is "a competent therapist using a bona fide therapy vetted in the peer-reviewed literature and through practice-based evidence drawing from the best available research while adjusting for individual and cultural differences and preferences with appropriate cultural humility" (p. 319).

Competencies are generalist, meaning they are basic knowledge, skills, and attitudes that all therapists must have. While they may be adapted to a degree by specific treatment modalities, all therapists, regardless of modality, should establish these competencies. Joel Vos (2025a) addresses these from an existential perspective.

Client characteristics, culture, and preference require therapists to be able to make adaptations based on individual and cultural differences and preferences. As illustrated consistently in this volume, adapting to individual differences and preferences is deeply integrated into the foundations of EH therapy and EH case formulation. Cultural differences, however, are more complex. In *The Evidence-Based Foundations of Existential–Humanistic Therapy* (Hoffman & Lac, 2025), there are chapters on most primary EH interventions, which are consistent with those identified in Chapter 2. In each of these chapters, cultural adaptations are considered. While there is a need for ongoing growth and development with cultural adaptations, these chapters demonstrate that EH therapy can make the necessary adjustments.

The best available research is controversial, partly because there is still a bias toward randomized clinical trials (RCTs) and meta-analyses, even though these are not always the best methodologies for investigating particular research questions (Hoffman, 2025). From an EH perspective, the research question should inform the methodology, which for outcome studies includes what is most appropriate for the modality. Allowing the question to determine the methodology is a foundational research competency that EBPP does not adhere to. Therefore, Hoffman recommended an amendment to understanding the best available research by shifting away from the bias toward certain approaches and, instead, focusing on the most appropriate methodology for the research question.

The chapters in *The Evidence-Based Foundations of Existential–Humanistic Therapy* (Hoffman & Lac, 2025) on specific interventions all include an overview of the research supporting them. While there are limitations, including that some of the research was not specifically on EH therapy outcomes, the overall results strongly demonstrate that there is clear empirical support for the foundations of EH therapy. This position has been affirmed by influential psychotherapy outcome researcher Bruce Wampold (2008).

In summary, the evidence supports EH therapy and its ability to be practiced consist with EBPP. In the rest of the chapter, we briefly address how the case formulation approach developed in this book can be used to demonstrate research support for the interventions. In addition, EH therapists must be able to demonstrate basic competencies and the ability to adapt their approach according to individual and cultural differences and preferences.

DEMONSTRATING RESEARCH SUPPORT FOR EXISTENTIAL–HUMANISTIC INTERVENTIONS IN THE TREATMENT PLAN

In RCTs, often touted as the gold standard, strict adherence to the therapy modalities is required, which rarely happens in the real world of therapy. Therefore, there is an inherent limitation built into RCTs that questions its status as the gold standard of best available research. Most therapists use integrative strategies, even if primarily adhering to one modality as a foundation. This is true of EH therapy as well, as demonstrated throughout this volume. Therefore, it is better to base research support on the stances and treatment interventions instead of outcome research focused on a rigid application of the therapy modality that does not match how it is practiced in the real world.

With the focus on the treatment intervention or stance, the approach to EH case formulation described in this book provides a solid foundation for demonstrating empirical support with approaches to individual clients. First, it is important that a specific treatment strategy or intervention is mapped onto one or more client goals. Second, research is cited supporting the effectiveness and/or efficacy of each intervention. *The Evidence-Based Foundations of Existential–Humanistic Therapy* (Hoffman & Lac, 2025) makes this easy. A shortcut would be simply to cite the relevant chapter from this book. This often is sufficient. However, a stronger approach is to cite the chapter and specific research within the chapter that is relevant to the particular intervention. Stronger yet, by keeping up with the relevant research on these interventions, new research not covered in Hoffman and Lac can also be included. EH therapists can save time by compiling a reference list of research articles and summaries supporting interventions in a document so they can easily cut and paste these into the individual treatment plans. These should be research articles or summaries of research, not theoretical articles.

In the following section, research support is cited for each EH intervention in Rasheeda's treatment plan.[1] Because these are already mapped with the client goals and cover each goal with at least one intervention, it demonstrates strong research support for Rasheeda's treatment plan. To save space, we cite the chapters from *The Evidence-Based Foundations of Existential–Humanistic Therapy* (Hoffman & Lac, 2025) and no more than two additional citations. Typically, three references should be sufficient.

---

[1]The case of Rasheeda is fictional and inspired by common themes and interactions with our clients.

EXAMPLE CASE FORMULATION FOR RASHEEDA: SUPPORT FOR TREATMENT APPROACHES, STANCES, AND/OR TECHNIQUES

Treatment Strategy 1

Presence will be used to strengthen the therapeutic relationship, cultivate deeper awareness, and increase relational depth.

Krug, O. T., Bradshaw, C., Ratner, J., & Sánchez-Mazarro, A. (2025). Therapeutic presence in existential–humanistic psychotherapy. In L. Hoffman & V. Lac (Eds.), *The evidence-based foundations of existential–humanistic therapy* (pp. 103–130). American Psychological Association. https://doi.org/10.1037/0000446-005

Geller, S. M., Greenberg, L. S., & Watson, J. C. (2010). Therapist and client perceptions of therapeutic presence: The development of a measure. *Psychotherapy Research, 20*(5), 599–610. https://doi.org/10.1080/10503307.2010.495957

Treatment Strategy 2

Self-disclosure was effective in early sessions to help develop a deeper therapy relationship and model self-disclosure to the client. Brief self-disclosures will continue to be used to model emotional expression and emotion management and facilitate relational depth.

Sebree, D., Jr., & Brown, V. (2025). Therapist self-disclosure in existential–humanistic psychotherapy. In L. Hoffman & V. Lac (Eds.), *The evidence-based foundations of existential–humanistic therapy* (pp. 293–310). American Psychological Association. https://doi.org/10.1037/0000446-013

Henretty, J. R., Currier, J. M., Berman, J. S., & Levitt, H. M. (2014). The impact of counselor self-disclosure on clients: A meta-analytic review of experimental and quasi-experimental research. *Journal of Counseling Psychology, 61*(2), 191–207. https://doi.org/10.1037/a0036189

Treatment Strategy 3

Vivification of protections will be used to increase awareness of how protections are impacting Rasheeda's relationships with other people.

Spaeth, D., Vanderhoff, J. A., Pintauro, M., & Hoffman, L. (2025). Authenticity, self-awareness, and facing life directly in existential–humanistic psychotherapy. In L. Hoffman & V. Lac (Eds.), *The evidence-based foundations of existential–humanistic therapy* (pp. 183–206). American Psychological Association. https://doi.org/10.1037/0000446-008

Treatment Strategy 4

Facilitating self-awareness will be used to help Rasheeda develop insight into relational patterns, including those that may be causing barriers to satisfying relationships. Facilitating self-awareness will also be used to help Rasheeda clarify values and what she is looking for in a romantic partner.

EXAMPLE CASE FORMULATION FOR RASHEEDA: SUPPORT FOR TREATMENT APPROACHES, STANCES, AND/OR TECHNIQUES (*Continued*)

Spaeth, D., Vanderhoff, J. A., Pintauro, M., & Hoffman, L. (2025). Authenticity, self-awareness, and facing life directly in existential–humanistic psychotherapy. In L. Hoffman & V. Lac (Eds.), *The evidence-based foundations of existential–humanistic therapy* (pp. 183–206). American Psychological Association. https://doi.org/10.1037/0000446-008

Sutton A. (2016). Measuring the effects of self-awareness: Construction of the Self-Awareness Outcomes Questionnaire. *Europe's Journal of Psychology, 12*(4), 645–658. https://doi.org/10.5964/ejop.v12i4.1178

Treatment Strategy 5

Here-and-now interventions will provide a foundation for increasing self-awareness in relationships and deepening emotional awareness.

Underwood, J. J. (2025). Here-and-now work in existential–humanistic psychotherapy. In L. Hoffman & V. Lac (Eds.), *The evidence-based foundations of existential–humanistic therapy* (pp. 207–224). American Psychological Association. https://doi.org/10.1037/0000446-009

Hill, C. E., Knox, S., & Pinto-Coelho, K. G. (2018). Therapist self-disclosure and immediacy: A qualitative meta-analysis. *Psychotherapy, 55*(4), 445–460. https://doi.org/10.1037/pst0000182

Treatment Strategy 6

The therapist's use of genuineness will be important for developing relational depth in the therapy relationship and facilitating the development of more genuine relationships outside of therapy.

Morrill, Z. (2025). Genuineness and the real relationship in existential–humanistic psychotherapy. In L. Hoffman & V. Lac (Eds.), *The evidence-based foundations of existential–humanistic therapy* (pp. 267–292). American Psychological Association. https://doi.org/10.1037/0000446-012

Kolden, G. G., Wang, C.-C., Austin, S. B., Chang, Y., & Klein, M. H. (2018). Congruence/genuineness: A meta-analysis. *Psychotherapy, 55*(4), 424–433. https://doi.org/10.1037/pst0000162

Treatment Strategy 7

Acceptance, genuineness, here-and-now explorations, and the facilitation of self-awareness will be used to address feelings of guilt and shame.

Morrill, Z. (2025). Genuineness and the real relationship in existential–humanistic psychotherapy. In L. Hoffman & V. Lac (Eds.), *The evidence-based foundations of existential–humanistic therapy* (pp. 267–292). American Psychological Association. https://doi.org/10.1037/0000446-012

(*continues*)

EXAMPLE CASE FORMULATION FOR RASHEEDA: SUPPORT FOR TREATMENT APPROACHES, STANCES, AND/OR TECHNIQUES (*Continued*)

Christensen, R., & Vincent, A. (2025). Understanding acceptance in existential-humanistic psychotherapy. In L. Hoffman & V. Lac (Eds.), *The evidence-based foundations of existential–humanistic therapy* (pp. 253–266). American Psychological Association. https://doi.org/10.1037/0000446-011

Underwood, J. J. (2025). Here-and-now work in existential–humanistic psychotherapy. In L. Hoffman & V. Lac (Eds.), *The evidence-based foundations of existential-humanistic therapy* (pp. 207–224). American Psychological Association. https://doi.org/10.1037/0000446-009

Treatment Strategy 8

Meaning-centered interventions will be used to address dissatisfaction and disconnection with important aspects of Rasheeda's life and promote general psychological well-being.

Vos, J. (2025b). Working with meaning in life in existential–humanistic psychotherapy. In L. Hoffman & V. Lac (Eds.), *The evidence-based foundations of existential-humanistic therapy* (pp. 225–252). American Psychological Association. https://doi.org/10.1037/0000446-010

Vos, J. (2018). *Meaning in life: An evidence-based handbook for practitioners.* Red Globe Press.

Treatment Strategy 9

The facilitation of emotional processing, acceptance, and empathy will be used for grieving Rasheeda's father's death and addressing emotions related to her sexual assault.

Varisco, B., & Hoffman, L. (2025). Working with emotions in existential–humanistic psychotherapy. In L. Hoffman & V. Lac (Eds.), *The evidence-based foundations of existential–humanistic therapy* (pp. 157–182). American Psychological Association. https://doi.org/10.1037/0000446-007

Christensen, R., & Vincent, A. (2025). Understanding acceptance in existential-humanistic psychotherapy. In L. Hoffman & V. Lac (Eds.), *The evidence-based foundations of existential–humanistic therapy* (pp. 253–266). American Psychological Association. https://doi.org/10.1037/0000446-011

Bohart, A. C., Shapiro, J. L, & Byock, G. (2025). Empathy in existential–humanistic psychotherapy. In L. Hoffman & V. Lac (Eds.), *The evidence-based foundations of existential–humanistic therapy* (pp. 131–156). American Psychological Association. https://doi.org/10.1037/0000446-006

DEMONSTRATING ONE'S PRACTICE IS CONSISTENT WITH EVIDENCE-BASED PSYCHOLOGICAL PRACTICE

With the research support demonstrated, EH therapists still must demonstrate basic competencies and the ability to adapt to individual and cultural differences. Competencies are difficult to demonstrate through a case formulation because these are basic skills that all professionals should maintain. Constructing a case formulation itself, however, demonstrates several of the competencies identified by the American Psychological Association, Presidential Task Force on Evidence-Based Practice (2006). EH therapists also demonstrate competencies by regularly participating in continuing education courses, staying current with relevant scholarly and research literature, engaging in critical reflection about one's practice, and using practice-based evidence.

Adapting to individual and cultural differences and preferences can be demonstrated throughout the case formulation. Many individualized factors are built into the EH case formulation and treatment progress, including identifying the client's perspective on the problem and client goals. Adapting to cultural differences and preferences can be identified and highlighted in how the case formulation is constructed through regularly attending to emerging cultural issues and discussing how these should impact treatment, including the adaptation of specific interventions.

CONCLUSION

Although those not familiar with EH therapy commonly assert that EH therapy does not fit with EBPP, it is easy for EH therapists to demonstrate that this is not accurate. In fact, EH therapy is on solid ground in adhering to the pillars of EBPP. In this chapter, we provided an overview of how EH therapists can use the case formulation template to support the research foundations of their work with individual clients.

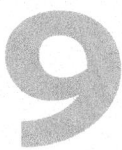

Additional Case Illustrations of Existential–Humanistic Case Formulation

This chapter has two additional examples of existential–humanistic (EH) case formulation.[1] With Rasheeda, a more extensive history illustrating how to translate from client history to the case formulation was included. The illustrations in this chapter are shorter and more focused. A brief history is followed by an example of the case formulation. The optional sections (i.e., diagnosis, alternate diagnosis, and treatment plans) and examples of how to use research to support the EH interventions are not included. Rather, the focus is on the EH-specific aspects of case formulation.

The example case formulations in this chapter do not provide a side-by-side comparison like Rasheeda's case formulations in previous chapters. However, they still demonstrate changes made over the course of 30 sessions. Text without any special formatting indicates information that was added through eight sessions. Bolded text indicates information that was added between Sessions 8 and 30, and crossed-out text indicates areas to follow up or clarify identified up to Session 8 that were integrated into the case formulation and omitted from their respective lists afterward.

---

[1]The case examples in this chapter follow fictional clients inspired by common themes and interactions with our clients.

https://doi.org/10.1037/0000464-010
Case Formulation in Existential–Humanistic Therapy, by L. Hoffman and H. P. Cleare-Hoffman

CASE ILLUSTRATION 1: HANK

The first case illustration in this chapter describes working with a client who presents quite differently than Rasheeda. Hank is a client who, at first glance, may seem like a client who would prefer a more solution-focused approach. However, as the case illustration demonstrates, an EH approach turned out to be a good fit.

Introduction to Hank

Hank is a 42-year-old, cisgender, heterosexual White male. After growing up in a small, Midwestern city, he attended a prestigious East Coast university. After graduation, he was hired as an executive in a growing tech company and steadily worked his way up to a vice president role by the time he was 33. After a few years in this role, he was informed that he was one of two people being considered for mentorship to become the company president when the founder retired. He worked hard and was selected for the role. Less than a year before he was to assume the role, the president met with him to apprise him that the company was being sold and that he would not become president after all. Hank was devastated and angry that he was not part of the decision to sell the company. He felt humiliated because he had been telling people that he would be president of the company by his 40th birthday. Hank began yelling at the president, leading to security being called. He calmed down but was still escorted out. Although Hank was supposed to have an upper leadership role at the new company, they decided not to retain him when they heard how he handled the news.

Expecting a big pay raise, Hank overextended himself and his family financially. He needed to find a job soon to meet his financial commitments, but word quickly spread about how he was fired, contributing to difficulty finding new employment. His wife, Camila, suggested they move to Colorado to be closer to her family. After resisting initially, Hank recognized this was the best option for their family. They sold their expensive home to get out of debt and began renting a modest home in Colorado. Although he was still unemployed when they moved, he was offered a job at a small nonprofit company that provided internet, computers, smartphones, and other technology to lower income families. He was overseeing a new division focused on providing training to the families receiving support with technology from the company. At first, he turned down the job because he did not think it was prestigious enough and felt he was overqualified. His wife convinced him to take the job and told him that it was an opportunity to return to the values they shared when they were first married.

Hank and Camila met in college. She was a first-generation college student from a Latinx family. When dating, they spoke of wanting to do something meaningful in the world. During the years Hank was an executive, their relationship became increasingly distant. Camila told Hank he had changed and become focused on money, power, and prestige. After they moved to Colorado, Camila admitted that she had been thinking of asking for a divorce for several years because of the changes in him. Hank became angry when Camila told him this and yelled, "Why did you make me move all the way to Colorado if you are just going to leave me!" Camila tried to tell him that this was a chance for a new start for them, too, but Hank refused to hear this.

After initial successes, Hank struggled at his new job. He was irritable and often snapped at people who reported to him. He was called into his supervisor's office and put on a performance improvement plan. He was told he had 6 months to develop more positive relationships with the people he was working with, or he would be demoted or let go. Hank considered quitting on the spot but worried that he did not have other options. He felt trapped. That night, he went to a bar with Vince, a colleague, and drank until he was quite intoxicated. He went to drive home, but Vince would not let him, taking his keys and calling Camila to pick him up.

The next day, Camila said that she and the children were going to stay with her parents for a while and implored Hank to get help. After she left, Hank briefly considered committing suicide. This shocked him because he had never had serious thoughts of suicide before. He called Vince and confessed he needed help. Vince recommended a therapist, Dr. M, who he immediately called. He set up an appointment with her.

Dr. M is a biracial psychologist in her mid-40s. When Hank met her, he was evidently surprised, which Dr. M suspected was because of her ethnicity. Noticing this, Dr. M reflected his reaction.

DR. M: You seemed surprised when we met. Tell me about that.

HANK: Yeah, well, I'm sorry. I guess I wasn't expecting [*trailing off*] . . .

DR. M: You weren't expecting to see a brown woman.

HANK: No, but I mean, it's okay. My wife, Camila, she's Latina. She'd probably say it's good for me. Maybe you can help me understand why Camila is so upset.

DR. M: Are you okay with this? It is important that we are both comfortable with the arrangements if we are going to work together.

HANK: I'm sorry. I am not making a good first impression, am I?

DR. M: To be honest, no. Do you want to see if we can turn it around?

HANK: Yes, I do. I mean, I will be better.

DR. M: Okay, I'm glad to hear that, but I also want you to be able to be yourself in here. I want you to be comfortable. Do you think that will be possible?

HANK: I think so. I'd like to give it a try. Like I said, maybe you can help me understand why Camila is so upset.

DR. M: Good. But let's check back in about this. Can you tell me what brought you in?

HANK: It has been a rough year. I had a great job and was in line to be the president of a large tech company on the East Coast. It all started when the company was being sold—I lost my temper and then lost my job. I mean, I was going to be president in less than a year, and they didn't even talk to me about it! Then, I couldn't get other employment, so we moved here to be near my wife's family. I found a job, but it is nothing like what I was doing. It's not fulfilling. Then I found out my wife has been thinking about leaving me for years. So, I went out last Friday to blow off some steam and got really drunk. My wife was pissed, took the kids, and has been staying with her parents. She told me to get help or she's leaving, so here I am.

DR. M: That's a lot in 1 year.

HANK: Yeah, and my life was great—perfect, really. I was making a boatload of money. I'd been moving up the ladder at work—everyone respected me. We were living the life. But now I'm here in a crappy job without my family and in therapy.

DR. M: It sounds like you're not happy about being here—in therapy—either.

HANK: Is anyone happy about needing to come to therapy?

DR. M: Fair point. Tell me about what you want to get from therapy.

HANK: I want to get my life back.

DR. M: What would that mean?

HANK: I want my wife and kids to move back in and get a better job so that my life can get back on track.

DR. M: Hmm. That's a challenging one. Those would be some difficult goals, and we don't have much control of that in here. What do you think would have to happen to accomplish these?

HANK: I don't know [*pausing*]. Isn't that what you're supposed to tell me?

DR. M: Maybe we can try to figure that out together.

HANK: I suppose . . . [*seeing Dr. M's reaction*]. I mean, yes.

This opening dialogue gives a sense of Hank's early presentation in therapy. Dr. M identified several markers for the therapy relationship, client motivation, and protections in this brief opening exchange. However, Dr. M approached these with some caution, working to avoid assumptions and keeping in mind that Hank was likely not comfortable coming to therapy for the first time.

Through the first eight sessions, Hank focused primarily on what happened at his job, particularly on feeling he was treated unfairly. Dr. M listened empathetically while encouraging him to reflect on his behavior. The primary problem Hank reported about himself was his alcohol consumption. He worried about this becoming more of a problem.

Sessions 9 to 30

In Sessions 9 to 22, progress was slow. Hank continued to focus on what happened to him, often putting himself in the victim role. He had three more episodes of drinking to the point of intoxication, which worried him, but both times, he drank less than before and was able to arrange for safe transportation home on his own.

In Session 22, Hank arrived dressed in a suit and tie. When Dr. M commented on this, he beamed, reporting that he had a job interview at a large tech company in Seattle shortly after the session. He was confident he would "blow them away" and get the job. In Session 23, he came in his regular work clothes, sat down, and began voicing frustrations with his current boss.

DR. M: Hank, I'm curious about what happened with the job interview.

HANK: I didn't get it.

DR. M: I'm really sorry, Hank. You were so excited and confident.

HANK: I thought it went well. After the interview, I told my wife I nailed it and was sure that I would get the job. That night, I started looking at realtors and houses in Seattle. Camila seemed worried that I was getting ahead of myself. I guess she was right. The next morning, I opened my email to the rejection letter. It didn't seem that I was even in the running. I didn't make it to the second round of interviews, not even close.

DR. M: Mm-hmm. [*Noticing some emotion, Dr. M paused with the silence.*]

HANK: Maybe it is me, after all. They didn't even get to references, so I can't blame what happened out East. . . . I guess part of me knew all along.

DR. M: It's hard to acknowledge.

HANK: Yeah, but you knew. You knew all along, didn't you? [*Pausing briefly, noticing the surprise in Dr M, and looking intently at her*] Come on, be honest—you knew?

DR. M: What would that mean to you?

HANK: [*Voice tone rising*] Come on, don't give me that BS. You're the one who keeps asking me about the relationship, and now you're dodging the question. You knew, didn't you?

DR. M: Fair enough. I try to always remember that I can't know for sure, but, yes, I have wondered about your contribution to the problems at your previous work. Rarely is it one-sided, and your anger caused you to do some things that made them concerned.

HANK: I knew you thought it—saw through me.

DR. M: Yet, you stuck with it.

HANK: I think I was trying to convince myself, too.

DR. M: That seems significant.

The rejection broke through some of Hank's protections. Over the next eight sessions, Hank increasingly began opening up, and the therapy progressed more quickly. He started showing more emotion, which mostly came out as anger at first. Gradually, he began acknowledging shame, sadness, and anxiety as well.

A few sessions after the rejection letter, he began acknowledging his role in his marital conflict, including discussing how he had changed from the person he was early in their marriage. He acknowledged that work had taken over as his priority, which often meant that his family came second. When he shared this with Camila, she began crying and hugged him. He reported feeling the tension decrease after this conversation, but he recognized many conversations were still needed.

Hank's performance at work improved just enough so that he was not fired or demoted; however, his supervisor told him they were going to continue the performance improvement plan for another 3 months. While disappointed and frustrated, this time, Hank was able to accept his responsibility and even acknowledge that keeping him on the performance improvement plan "might be fair."

In the following case formulation, we review Hank at eight and 30 sessions. Hank often avoided discussing many topics in depth early in therapy, leading to limited information from which to draw. This continued until Session 22, when Hank gradually began opening up more.

Brief Holistic Client Narrative

Hank was on track to become a successful executive in a technology firm. He described being happy with his life before it was derailed. The opening narrative gives a picture of the life he was living before he had significant problems at work, which was the type of life he wanted to return to when first entering therapy.

EXAMPLE CASE FORMULATION FOR HANK: BRIEF HOLISTIC CLIENT NARRATIVE

Hank is a 42-year-old male who has been married to Camila for 19 years. They have three children, a 13-year-old daughter, a 10-year-old son, and an 8-year-old daughter. He began dating Camila in his junior year at a prestigious university. He reported that when they first met, he would not have imagined dating her;

EXAMPLE CASE FORMULATION FOR HANK: BRIEF HOLISTIC CLIENT NARRATIVE (*Continued*)

however, after becoming friends, an attraction emerged. They shared many interests and values, particularly a dream to have a positive impact on people and the world around them.

After graduation, Hank was recruited to an entry-level executive position at a growing tech company. He became close with a senior-level administrator, Ross, who mentored him and encouraged him to prioritize advancement. Hank began working long hours and attending many conferences and training events. He quickly advanced to senior-level positions and was selected to be the next president before the company was sold, resulting in him looking for a new job and his family relocating to Colorado.

Early in their marriage, Hank and Camila were involved in various community projects and volunteered for a homeless shelter and disadvantaged children. He found meaning in what they were doing and doing it with Camila. He also enjoyed bicycling, skiing, and traveling. Since his late 20s, Hank has spent less time volunteering and on his hobbies.

In college, Hank was active socially and developed several close friendships with other men. Most of these friends have gone on to become business executives. Each year, they get together for a long weekend in Vermont to go skiing and catch up. While this group has been a source of encouragement and support, their friendships are also competitive. Hank enjoyed the competitive aspect of the friendships and took great pride in advancing more quickly than most of his friend group.

Concern or Problem Identification

Hank's life was derailed following a surprise transition at work that he did not handle well. The problem identification illustrates how this derailment began to illuminate other problems he was unaware of, such as his wife's marital dissatisfaction. Hank repressed, denied, or remained unaware of these difficulties at the outset of therapy.

EXAMPLE CASE FORMULATION FOR HANK: CONCERN OR PROBLEM IDENTIFICATION

Client's Description of the Concern or Problem

Initial Client Perspective on the Concern or Problem

In the first session, Hank reported that his problems were not having a job that fit his career aspirations and his wife, Camila, temporarily separating from him.

(continues)

EXAMPLE CASE FORMULATION FOR HANK: CONCERN OR PROBLEM IDENTIFICATION (*Continued*)

Since this time, Camila and their children have moved home, but he reports the conflict remains, and Camila warns him that if things do not improve, she will leave again. Hank describes himself as "upset" about what happened to him over the last year, which has led to a general irritability. He describes himself as often "short" with people at work and his family at home. Although he has more time for some of his hobbies now, he rarely engages in them and reports being uninterested in them. Since moving to Colorado, Hank "went on binges" four times and got intoxicated, which he reported he had never done before. Initially, he denied this was a concern, but as it happened more times, he began to worry about it becoming a pattern.

Emergent Client Perspective on the Concern or Problem

Hank eventually reported feeling guilty about his behavior that led to him getting fired, including acknowledging that if he were in the president's shoes, he would have fired him as well. However, he feels he went too far in telling other tech companies what happened, making it difficult to find a new job. Hank recognizes that he has changed in his relationship with Camila, including his priorities. He feels guilt about his behavior at work and the changes in his priorities and marriage. He believes the changes in him are the primary reason he feels more disconnected from his wife, children, and in-laws.

Areas to Follow Up or Clarify

- ~~There are markers suggesting Hank feels loneliness and isolation; however, when asked about this, he denied it.~~

- **While Hank has begun exploring and clarifying feelings of isolation from his family, he has not given much attention to his long-term friendships yet. He described his coworker Vince as becoming a closer friend.**

- Several markers suggest that Hank is no longer engaged with life, particularly his mentioning several times that he does not enjoy past hobbies. **There has been mild progress on this over the last few sessions.**

Diagnosis of Systems or Contextual Issues Impacting Psychological Health

Hank was recently fired and unable to find a new job where he was living. He did not want to move to Colorado, but he did because he could not find a job, and his wife insisted they move somewhere more affordable and closer to family because of their financial situation. Hank had overextended himself by acquiring a nice home, a vacation home, and expensive cars for his wife and himself before losing his job. They were able to pay off most of their debt by selling their home and vacation home, but they still have debt that is causing stress and contributing to conflict with his wife.

EXAMPLE CASE FORMULATION FOR HANK: CONCERN OR PROBLEM IDENTIFICATION (*Continued*)

Implications of the Concern or Problem

Hank lost his job after becoming angry and yelling at the company president when he was informed the company would be sold. He struggled to find another job. During this time, he began experiencing increased marital conflict. His wife told him she had not been happy in their marriage for many years before he lost his job, but more recently, she left with her children for about 2 weeks. When she moved home, it was conditional on him remaining in therapy and being more involved with their family again. Hank spends less time with his friends, including skipping a "guys trip" with close friends for the last several years. Hank was written up at his new job due to his poor treatment of people who report to him. He is not happy at his job, which leads to decreased motivation.

Legal and Ethical Issues

Hank had a brief period in which he considered suicide after his wife and children moved out. He denied any suicidal ideation since that night; however, this should be monitored. Hank rarely drank to the point of intoxication before moving to Colorado but has "binged" four times in the last year. On two of these occasions, he was going to drive home, and a friend or bartender stopped him.

Theoretical Aspects of the Case Formulation

Hank's reasons for being in therapy and his openness to exploring his contributions to the problems shifted significantly over the course of therapy. Initially, Hank blamed external factors for most of his problems. As he engaged the therapy process, he started to take more responsibility, which shifted the focus of therapy and his view of the issues he was facing. Hank's case illustration demonstrates why it is important to maintain a fluid approach to case formulation.

EXAMPLE CASE FORMULATION FOR HANK: THEORETICAL ASPECTS OF THE CASE FORMULATION

Client Strengths and Resources

Hank is intelligent and had a successful career in which he quickly advanced before being fired. When in a job that he likes, he is highly motivated. Hank has friends who are supportive of him, even after the loss of his job. His parents and brother have remained supportive of him through his challenges.

(continues)

EXAMPLE CASE FORMULATION FOR HANK: THEORETICAL ASPECTS OF THE CASE FORMULATION (*Continued*)

Areas to Follow Up or Clarify

Hank does not currently experience his wife as supportive; however, there are some indications she is trying to be supportive.

Biological and Physical Considerations

Hank reports that his blood pressure has increased since losing his job. His sleep patterns have been inconsistent, and he has not exercised as much over the past year. Otherwise, he reports being in good health.

Areas to Follow Up or Clarify

- Hank has not found a primary care physician or had a physical since moving to Colorado. **He actively avoided finding a primary care physician for a while but recently agreed to find one and schedule a physical.**

Family and Social Considerations

Hank grew up in a close, supportive family. His parents remained married. He had one younger brother, to whom he has always been close. He is part of a group of eight friends from college who have stayed in close contact, including getting together for a ski trip once a year. After getting fired, Hank skipped the next two ski trips, saying he could not afford them. He has not spoken with his friends often in the past 2 years, but they still send him encouragement.

Hank believed he had a good relationship with Camila until after moving to Colorado. However, she recently disclosed that she had not been happy in their marriage for several years, noting that he had changed. She complained he became focused on work, money, and power instead of the values that brought them together, **which he has acknowledged is accurate.** He gradually withdrew from the volunteer and service work they used to do together. Since moving, they have argued more frequently; **however, he reports the conflict has decreased since he started taking responsibility for his contributions to the marital conflict.** Before he lost his job, he said he had a good relationship with his wife's family. Since they moved, he has often skipped family events, saying he feels judged for having lost his job and not providing better for his family. Even though Camila insists her family has never judged him, Hank still believes it to be true.

Hank reported a "decent" relationship with his children but notes they are all closer to Camila. **He feels guilty for not being more active in his children's lives and believes this has led to not being as close to them as he would like.**

In recent months, Hank reported developing a deeper relationship with Vince, a colleague at work. Vince is his only close friend in Colorado outside of his family.

EXAMPLE CASE FORMULATION FOR HANK: THEORETICAL ASPECTS OF THE CASE FORMULATION (*Continued*)

Areas to Follow Up or Clarify

- There are markers suggesting that Hank believes others are judging him more than is true.

- Hank appears to have withdrawn from many of his long-term friendships, which may contribute to feelings of loneliness. **Several markers suggest this may be related to feelings of embarrassment and shame.**

- ~~Various markers suggest Hank has conflicting feelings about his role in the problems in his marriage. At times, he is critical of himself, while at other times, he uses language suggesting he sees himself as a victim.~~

- Hank quickly moves away from discussing Camila's family when they come up. He briefly noted feeling judged by them and not attending several family events with them.

- I am curious about Hank's feelings about being in a biracial relationship. He had some initial reaction that appeared to be related to me being a person of color and commented that his wife was initially not someone he would have imagined dating.

School and Employment Considerations

Hank was successful in his career until a little over a year ago when he was fired after becoming angry and yelling at his boss. After being fired, it was difficult to find another job until moving to Colorado. He reported not being happy in his current employment and feeling unmotivated. Hank was recently written up due to conflict with peers at his current job, which led to a night of drinking to the point of intoxication and an argument with his wife. **Hank recently had an interview for a job he was confident he would get, but he was not offered the position. Hank is beginning to identify aspects of his behavior that have contributed to problems at work.**

Areas to Follow Up or Clarify

- Hank has been unclear about what he is looking for in a career, typically stating that he wants to be successful or advance in his career, but he struggles to clarify what that means. Various markers suggest that his priority is a better paying, more prestigious job in an upper administrative role with some power or authority. **This seems to be shifting according to preliminary markers.**

(continues)

EXAMPLE CASE FORMULATION FOR HANK: THEORETICAL ASPECTS OF THE CASE FORMULATION (*Continued*)

Cultural Considerations

Hank is a White male married to a Latina woman. Hank comes from an upper-middle-class family, while Camila comes from a family that struggled with poverty.

Areas to Follow Up or Clarify

- Hank has not spoken much about being in an interracial marriage and having biracial children. He typically quickly downplays this and shifts the topic when something relevant is being discussed.

- It appears Hank has been influenced by his European heritage, including being socialized to the standards of White masculinity that have emerged more during his previous employment at the tech company. This may be contributing to his conflict with his wife.

- Hank appeared to have an initial negative reaction to me, which appeared to be related to me being a woman of color. He apologized for this but avoided talking about it. **Some markers suggest he may sometimes be cautious about what he says, though he generally has denied this when asked.**

Systemic Issues

There are no significant systemic issues identified other than those addressed in the employment section.

Areas to Follow Up or Clarify

- Hank has shifted away from conversations and topics that may connected with systemic issues, including the impact of being part of a biracial family.

Self-Awareness and Motivation

Hank avoided several topics early on, including potential family conflict and conflict at his current place of employment. He focused primarily on wanting there to be changes externally, particularly in his marriage and career. **This is gradually beginning to change, with Hank considering personal changes he would like to make, including concerns about his binge drinking, his "irritability" with his wife and people at work, and ways he contributes to conflicts in his marriage. Frank has begun reconsidering his values and priorities, including reclaiming values and priorities that he "fell away from."**

Hank is becoming increasingly open to reflections on his nonverbals and body language, though this is still new. He recognizes some of his nonverbal communication on his own, although this does not often happen yet.

EXAMPLE CASE FORMULATION FOR HANK: THEORETICAL ASPECTS OF THE CASE FORMULATION (*Continued*)

Areas to Follow Up or Clarify

- ~~It is not clear whether Hank's avoidance of topics may be related to protections, lack of self-awareness, or other possible reasons.~~

- ~~Hank initially appeared surprised by reflections of emotions and body language; he often paused and then sometimes changed the direction of the conversation. When I reflected this or tried to refocus on the previous topic, he continued to change the direction of the conversation.~~

Here-and-Now

Until the last eight sessions, Hank did not stay in the here-and-now long with personal reflection or the relational aspects of the here-and-now, consistently switching topics within a few seconds. **Hank is gradually becoming more comfortable with the here-and-now both intrapersonally and interpersonally, including initiating a couple of here-and-now discussions relevant to the therapy relationship.**

Areas to Follow Up or Clarify

- Some markers suggest that Hank may typically avoid the here-and-now in most relationships, not just therapy.

Existential Givens

Death and Finiteness

Hank said that he does not feel significant since losing his job; he feels others, particularly in-laws and former colleagues, look down on him. He also feels that people at his new job do not respect him, contributing to feelings of insignificance. **He worries that he lost Camila's respect when he lost his job. They have begun talking about this. While she acknowledges that she lost some respect for him, it was because he was no longer involved in volunteer work and less involved with his family. She was hopeful when he lost his job that it may have been an opportunity to refocus on values they shared early in their marriage. Hank is beginning to see this as an opportunity as well, though he has not made any changes beyond discussing this with his wife and in therapy.**

Areas to Follow Up or Clarify

- ~~While Hank has not stated it directly, some markers suggest that he may worry Camila and his children also have lost respect for him from losing his job.~~

(*continues*)

EXAMPLE CASE FORMULATION FOR HANK: THEORETICAL ASPECTS OF THE CASE FORMULATION (*Continued*)

- **Some markers suggest that Hank may still worry that many people, including his children, in-laws, and possibly his college friends, may have lost respect for him.**

Freedom, Responsibility, and Agency

Since losing his job, Hank reported feeling "powerless" and "not having control" over various aspects of his life, including his career, his relationship with his wife, and his relationship with his friends. He described this as feeling trapped. **Initially, he blamed this on other people. Recently, he began acknowledging his responsibility for what transpired at both jobs.**

Areas to Follow Up or Clarify

- Hank tends to use language suggesting that he sees himself as a victim in losing his job, not being able to get a new job, and being written up at his new job.

- When Hank sees himself as a victim, he tends to avoid engagement. For example, he avoided talking with people he believes are judging him.

- Various markers suggest that Hank does not recognize the choices he is making or avoiding making, such as believing he does not have a choice in career direction. **This has improved, but the pattern continues in some areas.**

- **There are markers suggesting that as Hank has begun taking responsibility for his contributions to work and marital conflicts, he is experiencing more freedom. This has not yet been confirmed with Hank.**

Relationships, Isolation, and Alienation

Hank withdrew from many of his close relationships, including relationships with his friends and some family members, after losing his job. Hank initially denied feeling lonely; **however, he recently began acknowledging feelings of isolation and loneliness.**

Areas to Follow Up or Clarify

- There are several markers of intrapersonal isolation, which may contribute to his experience of isolation. These include not acknowledging, even to himself, mistakes he made contributing to conflict at work and with Camila.[2]

---

[2]This area to follow up or clarify has been addressed in the Self-Awareness and Motivation section.

EXAMPLE CASE FORMULATION FOR HANK: THEORETICAL ASPECTS OF THE CASE FORMULATION (*Continued*)

- ~~When Hank talks about his relationships, the descriptions tend to fit better with isolation than loneliness.~~

- Hank often suggests that he does not need many friends; however, historically, his descriptions are of having a large friend group.

Emotions and Embodiment

At the beginning of therapy, Hank used vague word choices for his emotions, such as feeling "irritable" or "off" or describing himself as being "short" with others. **He still primarily uses these words but has begun discussing feeling embarrassment, guilt, and shame. Hank has begun acknowledging his anger, too. As he has done this, his anger has decreased.** In early sessions, Hank's emotions were contained, not showing many emotions. **He began being more open with his emotions in sessions recently.**

Areas to Follow Up or Clarify

- ~~When I try to explore emotions with Hank, he often avoids typical emotional language. It is not clear if this may be a protection, reflect a limited emotional vocabulary, or be due to other factors. Early markers suggest clarifying that this may be a slow process with Hank.~~

Meaning

At the beginning of therapy, Hank reported that his family was his central priority. He initially denied that work and his role at work was important, suggesting instead that he was focused on his career to "provide a good life" for his family. **Hank now acknowledges that his values and priorities have shifted since he was in college and his first years of marriage to Camila. He is considering what reclaiming his values and priorities may look like and if he wants to pursue this more. Concerning his acknowledgment of value changes, he admitted that an upper-management role at a company has been important to him and still is, though he is rethinking this.**

Areas to Follow Up or Clarify

- ~~Hank denies that work, including being in a leadership role, is important to him when discussing the topic directly and, instead, indicates he wants a successful career to give his family "whatever they want." However, his career is the primary topic he focuses on in therapy, and when I try to explore other topics, he typically quickly shifts back to this topic.~~

(continues)

EXAMPLE CASE FORMULATION FOR HANK: THEORETICAL ASPECTS OF THE CASE FORMULATION (*Continued*)

Daimonic

Hank reported concern about his drinking habits as of late, which includes four occasions of drinking to the point of intoxication in the last year—something he rarely did before moving to Colorado. **As he has shifted to focusing on other issues, he reports being less worried about his drinking and notes that his desire to drink has substantially subsided. Hank acknowledges that he had become consumed with advancement and wealth, which had been driving his behaviors. He would still like to have a better job with an upper management position and the potential for advancement and better pay, but he is beginning a process of clarifying and reassessing his values and priorities related to this.**

Areas to Follow Up or Clarify

- ~~Several markers suggest that Hank has been consumed by a desire for career advancement, power, and wealth.~~

Self-Acceptance

Hank initially gave mixed reports about his acceptance of himself. Regarding his work and marriage, he mostly spoke positively of himself. **As therapy progressed, he has been more critical of himself, including reporting embarrassment, guilt, and shame.** He reported disappointment in himself and concerns about his drinking early in therapy. **Now, he reports less concern about his drinking and is embarrassed about having turned to alcohol to cope. At the beginning of therapy, he did not** believe he should have been fired and described strong confidence in his ability and value to a company. **More recently, he acknowledged he would have fired himself, too, if he was in his boss's shoes.**

Areas to Follow Up or Clarify

- ~~Hank gives unclear messages pertaining to self-acceptance. Most frequently, he speaks highly of himself and demonstrates defensiveness. However, at times, he is briefly critical of himself. This seems to be gradually shifting.~~

- **Hank's self-acceptance appears, on the surface, to be going in the wrong direction. However, this is likely connected to accepting his responsibility, which may reflect a stage in the change process.**

Client-Therapist Relationship

Hank **was** hesitant in the therapy relationship, particularly addressing the here-and-now **early in therapy**. He often stammered, avoided eye contact when discussing the therapy relationship, and quickly changed topics. **This has begun changing; however, the change is gradual, with some points of hesitation remaining.**

EXAMPLE CASE FORMULATION FOR HANK: THEORETICAL ASPECTS OF THE CASE FORMULATION (*Continued*)

Areas to Follow Up or Clarify

- Hank initially appeared to be uncomfortable with his therapist being a woman of color. As Hank avoided the here-and-now, this was difficult to assess. **More recently, some markers suggest this is decreasing if it was present. Hank may be more open to exploring this now.**

Therapist's Perspective on the Client–Therapist Relationship

The therapy relationship with Hank developed slowly for the first 6 months. **More recently, it has begun to develop more steadily. It is still early in this transition. Due to Hank's difficulties with discussing the here-and-now, it has been difficult to assess the therapy relationship. As this improves, it may become easier to assess over the next several months.**

Treatment Planning

Hank's desired therapy outcome significantly evolved over the course of therapy, which is a common occurrence. This illustrates well why it is important to continue to help clients clarify their goals over the course of therapy. When the initial goals are rigidly adhered to without ongoing consideration, it can limit the therapy process.

EXAMPLE CASE FORMULATION FOR HANK: TREATMENT PLANNING

Narrative of the Client's Desired Outcome

Hank described wanting a job with a better salary that "reflects his abilities and potential." He described wanting his wife, children, and in-laws to respect him. In his marriage, Hank would like more "mutual support," which includes his wife accepting him, supporting his career goals, and speaking well of him with her family. Hank would like to return to going on ski trips with his friends after having a job that "better reflects who he is."[3]

(continues)

---

[3]As Hank's desired outcomes for treatment have changed significantly, the original paragraph can be deleted and replaced with the following paragraph.

EXAMPLE CASE FORMULATION FOR HANK: TREATMENT PLANNING (*Continued*)

Hank's vision of what he would like life to be like after therapy is evolving. He would like a closer relationship with his wife, similar to how it was early in their marriage. Hank would also like to feel closer to his children and feel that he has their respect. While his career is still important to him, he is rethinking his values related to his career. He is also rethinking his disengagement from volunteer work and many of his hobbies. Hank would like to begin participating in the ski trips with his friends again.

Areas to Follow Up or Clarify

- Hank's thoughts of what he would like life to look like after therapy have been rapidly evolving. Because it is in a state of transition, many aspects of this need continued attention.

Initial Client Goals

- no more alcohol binges

- improve marital relationship with less conflict and more support

- obtain a new job in which he is happier and more satisfied. **Hank is reconsidering this goal; he now feels that his current job could be a good fit if he can improve his work relationships.**

Emergent Client Goals

- clarify and engage in more meaningful activities, including activities that involve his wife
- develop a closer relationship with his children and in-laws
- face his fear of being judged by his friends and discuss with them more honestly what happened when he was fired
- decrease anger and irritability with colleagues and family
- develop better work relationships at his current job

Anticipated Challenges and/or Barriers

The client's goals and focus include many aspects that are hard to control because they are influenced by outside factors, including other people. It has been difficult to refocus the client on more realistic goals. The client is not happy living in Colorado and not happy with his current job. In general, he tends to avoid taking responsibility for his behaviors, often blaming others.[4]

---

[4]Because barriers and challenges to treatment with Hank have changed significantly, the original paragraph can be deleted and replaced with the following paragraph.

EXAMPLE CASE FORMULATION FOR HANK: TREATMENT PLANNING (*Continued*)

The client has recently shifted his focus for therapy and the directions he wants to pursue in life. This is a recent change; therefore, some previous barriers could return.

Areas to Follow Up or Clarify

- The client's motivation for personal change appears to be mixed, and his self-awareness appears to be mixed. **This is beginning to change by reflecting more motivation and awareness.**

- **As the client's desired direction in life and therapy is clarified, it will be important to reassess for new potential challenges and/or barriers.**

Existential–Humanistic Treatment Strategies and Interventions

- vivification and working with protections. This is targeting his relational conflicts, drinking, and barriers to getting a better job.

- presence to facilitate self and interpersonal exploration to address relational conflict

- facilitation of self-awareness, searching strategies, and meaning-oriented interventions to clarify and engage in more meaningful activities

- acceptance and here-and-now interventions to facilitate improved relational awareness, improved relationships with family and close friends, and preparation for addressing worries about his friend's perceptions

- facilitation of emotional processing to address anger issues

- **genuineness, including sensitively providing feedback and facilitating the development of genuineness in relationships with others**

- **here-and-now interventions to facilitate moving toward more genuine relationships in which he is honest and vulnerable with friends and family. This also will address his fear of being judged.**

Integrative Strategies

- mindfulness strategies to promote emotional and interpersonal awareness and acceptance of his emotions
- incorporation of breathing strategies for managing anger

(*continues*)

EXAMPLE CASE FORMULATION FOR HANK: TREATMENT PLANNING (*Continued*)

Treatment Progress

Hank's progress was slow through the first 6 months of therapy. Since then, there has been a noticeable shift, with progress occurring more rapidly. Hank has demonstrated improved self-awareness and vulnerability in sessions. As this has been discussed in therapy, he also began being more vulnerable in his marriage, which has led to a decrease in marital conflict. He reported that temptations for binge drinking have completely subsided; however, this has been recent, so it is not clear if it will continue. Hank's irritability and anger have decreased, particularly toward people. This has contributed to decreased conflict at home and, to a lesser degree, at work. It may take longer for an improvement at work. Hank began reconsidering engaging in meaningful activities and hobbies that were important to him for much of his life. He is reconsidering the job that he would like as well. While he still hopes to find a different job, he is less focused on upper administrative roles and higher pay. He also reports believing he could be happy at his current job if the people he has not treated well can forgive him, and he is able to build more positive relationships with colleagues.

CASE EXAMPLE 2: JACINTA

Jacinta had been through many difficult times before entering therapy, including the loss of her husband, major life transitions, and encounters with racism. However, what prompted her to begin therapy was an unexpected reaction when a man she was getting to know asked her on a date. The case illustrates working with powerful, unexpected emotions connected to prior unresolved life events.

Introduction to Jacinta

Jacinta is a 36-year-old cisgender Latina woman and a widowed mother with two children. She is originally from Albuquerque, New Mexico. Jacinta's oldest son, Daniel, is 13. His father is her college boyfriend, Greg, a White man who became emotionally abusive and tried to talk her into an abortion after she became pregnant. Daniel has never met his father or any members of his father's family. Jacinta met her husband, Gabriel, when Daniel was 3. They married, and he adopted Daniel. They have another son, Emilio, who is now 7. Four years ago, Gabriel was killed in an accident at work due to improper safety measures at the plant where he worked. After Gabriel died, Jacinta received a modest settlement from his employer and moved to Colorado to get away from the bad memories in Albuquerque. Many members of her family live in Colorado, which is why she chose to move there. With the settlement money, Jacinta opened a store selling products made in Latin America and the Caribbean.

When she first moved to Colorado, Jacinta entered therapy for grief related to her husband's death. She reported learning a few skills to manage her emotions but did not feel therapy overall was helpful. She has not been in therapy since. Jacinta's store has been successful; however, her landlord ended the lease because he was concerned about meetings that she was holding at the store. After her husband's death, Jacinta was convinced that there were poor safety measures at his work because the company hired mostly immigrants and undocumented workers who she believes they saw as unlikely to complain about working conditions. Her concern about this led her to join a couple of advocacy groups that she allowed to meet for free in the backroom of her store. Gradually, she became more involved with the groups, including taking on a leadership role. Her landlord alleged that she was engaging in illegal behavior, claiming that some people attending the meetings were undocumented. Jacinta did not know if this was true and, not wanting to risk getting anyone in trouble, did not fight back at being asked to leave. With the help of her family and some people in the meetings, she was able to get a loan to purchase her own building with ample space for her store and a larger space for meetings in the back. She also converted a fenced-in area behind the store into a playground for neighborhood children.

Six months ago, Jacinta met Bruce. He began frequenting her store, often staying around to talk for longer periods. When Bruce found out about one of the meetings, he asked if he could attend. Jacinta agreed. Bruce was the only White man at the meeting but became a regular and fit in well. One month ago, Bruce asked Jacinta to go on a date with him. She did not anticipate her reaction when Bruce asked her out. Immediately, she began having intense anxiety, building to a panic attack, and then began crying. She did not understand her emotions. Bruce calmly tried to comfort her. When she looked at him, his eyes were welling up with tears. Worried she hurt him, she said, "I'm sorry. I'm just not ready for this. I need some time and space." Bruce left, apologizing and asking her to call if he could help. Later, he texted her check to see if she was okay, and a few days later asked if it was still okay for him to come to the meetings. Jacinta responded, asking him to give her some time before attending again. Bruce agreed and began texting about once a week to ask how she was doing, but he continued to respect her boundaries.

Sessions 1 to 8
Jacinta decided to give therapy another try, this time intentionally seeking out a therapist who was a woman of color. As she called therapists, she specifically stated she did not just want to learn how to cope with emotions.

After speaking to a few therapists, she scheduled an appointment with Dr. C, a Black cisgender woman, for an initial consultation.

DR. C: Jacinta, tell me what brings you in.

JACINTA: I didn't think I would ever come back to therapy. . . . I'm sorry. I'm a bit nervous.

DR. C: It's okay to be nervous. Many people are when they first come in. It sounds like you had a bad experience in therapy before.

JACINTA: Not really. I mean, it was fine. It just wasn't very helpful. Well, that's not right [*appearing increasingly nervous*]. I mean, I learned some things that have helped with my emotions, but it just wasn't what. . . . I'm not sure.

DR. C: Take your time, Jacinta. Maybe take a breath.

JACINTA: Yes, that's what I learned before [*taking a breath*].

DR. C: Don't worry, that's not all we are going to do here. But it might help you settle in a bit.

JACINTA: [*Looking slightly calmer*]

DR. C: Okay, are you ready to begin?

JACINTA: Yes. My husband died a few years ago, and I have not dated since then. Then this guy, Bruce, started coming into my store. He is nice, sweet, and good-looking. We started getting to know each other. I could tell he liked me, so I figured it was coming, but when he finally asked me out, all these emotions overtook me [*eyes filling with tears*]. I was anxious and having trouble breathing, but mostly, I just felt all this sadness. I asked him to leave and told him that I needed space.

DR. C: It is still a lot, even just talking about it in here.

JACINTA: Yes. I don't know why. . . . I just want to know why.

DR. C: Why the emotions were so intense?

JACINTA: Yes. I've never had a panic attack before, but I think this was one. I've been through stuff much worse, so why would I have a panic attack now? When a nice guy asks me out?

DR. C: I don't know, but I think we can figure it out together.

As the session progressed, Jacinta's anxiety decreased, but she continued having periods of sadness and crying. Dr. C intentionally inquired about aspects of her life beyond the event with Bruce to provide some space from Bruce in therapy as well, which helped Jacinta feel more comfortable. When Dr. C asked what she would like from therapy, she kept saying that she wanted to understand why she reacted the way she did. Toward the end of the session, Dr. C shared her approach to therapy, including introducing EH therapy in nontechnical jargon, particularly emphasizing the relationship and working with emotions. Dr. C also clarified the difference between solution-focused and depth approaches, noting that she belonged more in the latter category. She then asked if Jacinta had any questions.

JACINTA: Yes. Can you tell me a bit about you?

DR. C: Okay, what would you like to know?

JACINTA: I just think I would feel more comfortable knowing a bit more about who you are. . . . I mean, not just your credentials and approach to therapy.

DR. C: I am happy to answer your question. I may be able to answer it a bit better if I knew why this would be helpful.

JACINTA: I'm not fully sure. I just know that I don't know who you are. I guess part of it is wanting to know if you can understand me. I mean, we are both women of color, but you're a doctor. And [*trailing off*] . . .

DR. C: I think I'm getting it. I'll give it a try, but let me know if this is not what you need. Okay?

JACINTA: Okay.

DR. C: I am one of those rare Colorado natives. I knew since high school that I wanted to be a therapist. I worked hard and was able to get scholarships for college and then graduate school, where I obtained my master's degree and then my first license. I worked hard again and went back to school to get my doctorate, and now I am a psychologist. I have a husband and three children. My husband is a teacher at a high school here in town. Is this helpful?

JACINTA: Yes. Your husband—is he also Black?

DR. C: Yes.

JACINTA: Oh [*sounding disappointed*].

DR. C: That didn't seem like the answer you were hoping for.

JACINTA: I'm not sure why, but I kind of hoped that you were in a biracial relationship.

DR. C: So I could relate to you?

JACINTA: Yes.

DR. C: I don't know if it helps, but I did date some men who were not Black when I was in college, including some serious relationships.

This provided some insight into the unique challenges biracial relationships sometimes encounter. And I work with many individuals and couples in multiracial relationships.

JACINTA: Yes, and it really shouldn't matter. I don't know why I asked.

DR. C: But right now, it does. That's okay. As we get to know each other, please let me know if concerns about this or about me being Black come up for you. It is important for us to discuss this.

JACINTA: Okay, I will.

In the first eight sessions, Jacinta was quite open with her emotions. Her primary focus was on what happened with Bruce. In particular, she worried that Bruce was hurt by her reaction to his asking her out and asking him to give her time and space. She also worried she was being unfair by asking him not to attend the meetings. In a couple of sessions, she discussed worries about health concerns at the beginning of the session. Dr. C recommended getting a physical after exploring Jacinta's anxiety about health issues. Jacinta noted that these had begun more recently. On a couple of occasions, Jacinta mentioned her husband and briefly mentioned that her first son was from a different relationship but did not say much about it. In Session 7, Dr. C reflected that each time Jacinta's husband came up, she became tearful. Jacinta began crying. With some exploration, Jacinta and Dr. C agreed that she had not grieved for her husband sufficiently, largely because she felt she needed to focus on her sons, the settlement, and then the move to Colorado.

Sessions 8 to 30

In Sessions 8 to 30, there was a steady progression of therapy, including the emergence of new themes. In Sessions 8 to 15, much of the focus was on grieving for her husband. On a couple of occasions, when focusing on grief, Dr. C's eyes welled up with tears. Each time, Jacinta apologized. After the second time this occurred, Dr. C responded.

DR. C: Jacinta, I am moved by your sadness, but you don't need to apologize for this.

JACINTA: I shouldn't put this on you. You're trying to help.

DR. C: Caring is part of trying to help. But I am curious what my tears mean to you.

JACINTA: That I am sharing too much or that I am causing you to be sad.

DR. C: I appreciate the sadness that I am feeling, Jacinta. The sadness is empathy, feeling with you. While there is sadness there, I also feel more connected to you when feeling the sadness. That balances out the sadness and can be helpful for our process in here.

JACINTA: Oh.

DR. C: I am curious about your reaction to what I shared.

JACINTA: I hadn't thought of it that way.

DR. C: Okay, that's your thoughts, though. I am also curious about any emotions that came up about what I shared.

JACINTA: I'm not sure.

DR. C: Take your time. Stay with it for a moment.

JACINTA: It's a bit uncomfortable. It's good in ways but also uncomfortable.

DR. C: Tell me more about that.

JACINTA: I am just not used to that. My family are all pretty emotional but not so much with sadness, except at funerals. And Gabriel . . . he was so calm and steady. This is new. It's a lot.

DR. C: Too much?

JACINTA: Maybe. It's just very intense. At times, maybe I need it, but it feels too much at times.

DR. C: Sounds like we may need to adjust the pace—slow it down sometimes. I will try to watch this, but I invite you to let me know anytime it feels too intense.

Dr. C was more cautious with her presence and empathy, recognizing the intensity Jacinta felt with this and checking in with Jacinta frequently. As Dr. C modulated this and checked in with Jacinta, Jacinta became more comfortable expressing more sadness and with Dr. C's empathetic responses, including tears.

In working with the grief, Jacinta, at times, became angry that Gabriel was not here to support her in what she was going through. This helped identify issues related to her store and the advocacy groups. She discussed receiving hate mail and occasional threats. She is not sure if this is because of the advocacy groups or because her store sells Latin American and Caribbean products. On a couple of occasions, she had graffiti sprayed on her store, saying, "Go back to Mexico" on her windows. She reported some anger about this, but fear tended to overwhelm the anger.

Bruce received less attention in Sessions 8 to 15. As Jacinta began focusing less on her grief, Bruce came up again in session 16. Again, Jacinta was worried that she hurt him by asking for space. Bruce continued to check in but less frequently. Right before Session 18, Bruce texted her for the first time in almost a month right before her session. After entering the office, Dr. C recognized something was happening. Dr. C began the session differently than she typically does.

DR. C: Jacinta, something seems different, just as you walked into the room.

JACINTA: I just got a text from Bruce. [*Several seconds of silence*] I don't know why, but it just brought up a lot. I didn't respond. I don't know how to respond.

DR. C: Tell me about that.

JACINTA: I just keep seeing his eyes, standing there with tears welling up and streaming down his face.

DR. C: We've talked about that before, but after our conversation, when you reacted to my tears. I am wondering if you have different thoughts about this.

JACINTA: [*Looking intently at Dr. C*] You mean he was just being empathetic?

DR. C: I don't know. I've never met Bruce. I wonder if that would change things.

JACINTA: [*Pausing, reflecting*] Maybe [*reflecting more*]. So maybe he was feeling connected to me, and I pushed him away.

DR. C: Let's stay with that first part for a minute. He was feeling connected to you.

JACINTA: [*Appearing anxious*]

DR. C: That brought up something different.

JACINTA: Yeah, I feel like I want to crawl out of my skin, but I don't know why.

DR. C: Is it too much? Are you able to stay with it?

JACINTA: Yeah, yeah. I can stay with it. [*Silence for several seconds, then shaking her head*]

DR. C: There was something there again.

JACINTA: My ex-boyfriend, Greg, Daniel's father, just popped into my head. But he was nothing like Bruce.

DR. C: Yet there seems to be a connection.

JACINTA: Maybe, but I don't know what [*appearing irritated*].

DR. C: There was another shift there.

JACINTA: I lost it—the feeling. It's gone. Now I'm just irritated that Daniel is stuck in my head. I don't like thinking about him.

The rest of the session, Jacinta struggled to get back in touch with her emotions. Dr. C encouraged her to journal about what happened in the session and after receiving the text from Bruce. After the session, while still in the lobby, Jacinta briefly responded to Bruce, thanking him for checking in and not giving up on her. In the next several sessions, Bruce and the advocacy groups were the primary focus. As Jacinta talked about Bruce, she began acknowledging that she wanted to give a relationship with him a try, but each time she came close to calling him, she "froze."

By Session 25, Jacinta no longer felt overwhelmed by the intensity of the sessions, which Dr. C and Jacinta discussed. She began appreciating and reciprocating the feelings of deep connection in the moments of empathy. She worried Bruce had moved on but still had not reached out to him and just gave brief responses when he texted her. She began discussing feeling more afraid about the hate messages that she received, even though they were less frequent. Dr. C noticed a pattern of the topics switching from Bruce to Greg to her shop and the hate messages.

DR. C: I've noticed that when we are talking about Bruce, Greg often comes up, and soon after, we start talking about the hate messages at your store.

JACINTA: I hadn't noticed that [*reflecting in silence*]. I haven't really talked much about what happened with Greg in here, just that it ended.

DR. C: It seems relevant now.

JACINTA: I think so. I knew Greg's family didn't approve of him dating a Brown girl. I had suspected it—whenever his family visited, he never introduced me to them. But he never said anything until I got pregnant. He told me that his family would never approve, and we had to have an abortion. I refused. He broke off the relationship and began sending me these angry messages, berating me. I thought our relationship was serious, but I realized I was just exotic and fun for him. He never intended for the relationship to be serious. I should have seen the signs. I was in denial. After I told him he didn't have to be involved—financially or helping to raise our son—he left me alone. We never spoke again.

DR. C: And now you are worried that you are in denial with Bruce.

JACINTA: [*Crying*] Yes.

As Jacinta made the connection between Bruce and Greg, she began focusing on how they were different. After a few weeks of discussing this, she texted Bruce, inviting him to stop by the store. When he did, she told him that she had been working through some things and that if Bruce were still interested and not dating anyone else, she would like to go on the date. Bruce had been on a couple of dates with other women but told Jacinta they did not go well, which he thought was because he was still interested in Jacinta. When they went on the date, she asked him to be patient and told him that going on a date brought up a lot of emotions. Bruce was patient and suggested they take things slow, which gave her more confidence.

In recent sessions, Jacinta began exploring her health anxiety. In earlier sessions, she and Dr. C recognized some connections with her husband's death, thinking this was the primary influencing factor. In recent sessions, markers emerged suggesting this is connected to being a single parent and fears of not being there for her children if she were to become sick or die. As Dr. C reflected on the markers, it became clearer to Jacinta that there was a strong connection with fears of abandoning her children due to health issues. While these fears remained, with the insight, she was better able to understand and manage the anxiety.

Brief Holistic Client Narrative

Jacinta's life was centered on her family, which had changed since the death of her husband and relocating to Colorado. She has been building a community with relatives and Latinx individuals and families.

EXAMPLE CASE FORMULATION FOR JACINTA: BRIEF HOLISTIC CLIENT NARRATIVE

Jacinta is a 36-year-old widowed mother of two children, Emilio and Daniel, ages 7 and 13. Jacinta's husband, Gabriel, who was also the father of Emilio, was a "great father and husband" but died several years ago in a work accident. Since his death, Jacinta relocated to Colorado and opened a store selling Latin American and Caribbean products. The store has been successful despite being targeted with hateful racial messages at times.

Jacinta has a good relationship with her sons, who are both doing well in school and extracurricular activities. They walk to her store together after school, often accompanied by friends with whom they play in the small, fenced-in playground behind the store. Jacinta developed close relationships with the parents of the other children, who appreciate them being able to hang out with her children in a safe place. Many of the parents also attend meetings at her store related to advocacy groups she hosts. These groups have been an important source of community and support.

Many of Jacinta's relatives, including aunts, uncles, and cousins, live nearby. They have many family gatherings, and several of her cousins attend the meetings at her store. Her cousins help at the store so Jacinta can attend events at her children's school. They also cover for her so that she can take vacations to Albuquerque to visit her parents and other relatives.

Recently, Jacinta began dating Bruce, the first person she has dated since the death of her husband. Although there were barriers to beginning to date again, Jacinta feels increasingly comfortable with Bruce and appreciates his willingness to move slowly. Jacinta and Bruce share many interests and values, and he has become engaged with the advocacy groups she hosts.

Concern or Problem Identification

Jacinta's identification of problems has various layers. While an event from shortly before beginning therapy prompted her to set up the appointment, her reaction to this event was connected to her husband's death and the experiences she had since moving to Colorado.

EXAMPLE CASE FORMULATION FOR JACINTA: CONCERN OR PROBLEM IDENTIFICATION

Client's Description of the Concern or Problem

Initial Client Perspective on the Concern or Problem

Jacinta became overwhelmed with emotions when Bruce asked her out on a date. Jacinta was surprised by this reaction and the emotions that continued for days. Her primary concern is understanding her reaction to being asked out by Bruce. Second, she wants to be able to manage these emotions better; however, she was clear even before beginning her first session that she did not just want to learn skills to manage emotions. Jacinta did not sufficiently grieve her husband's death, partially due to being focused on taking care of her children, managing a settlement from her husband's employer, and moving to Colorado. Last, Jacinta experiences distress from hateful racial messages sent to her store and, at times, not feeling safe due to this.

Emergent Client Perspective on the Concern or Problem

Jacinta recognized that she is still experiencing emotional distress from a painful relationship with her oldest son's father, Greg, who she dated in college. While Jacinta has a good social support network, she does not always use it well for some of her needs. She has felt "alone" with aspects of her suffering, particularly areas of sadness and worry about her children.

Areas to Follow Up or Clarify

- A lack of clarity regarding Jacinta's reaction to Bruce asking her out on a date remains. There appears to be a connection with the death of her husband that we have discussed, but there also appears to be more to it that has not been identified yet.

Diagnosis of Systems or Contextual Issues Impacting Psychological Health

Jacinta recently was forced to move her business due to her landlord's concern about her involvement with advocacy groups meeting in the back of her store. Initially, she was angry about this and was going to fight having to move,

(continues)

EXAMPLE CASE FORMULATION FOR JACINTA: CONCERN OR PROBLEM IDENTIFICATION (*Continued*)

but he accused her of having people who "are here illegally" at the meetings. She did not know if this was true, having never inquired about immigration status, so she decided to move to prevent people at the meetings encountering difficulties. While she was able to purchase a building with the support of family and friends, this increased her stress due to financial worries about the store. She continues to receive hate messages at her building on occasion, which causes anxiety and fear for her and her children's safety. She is also angry that the police have not done more to investigate and stop this.

Implications of the Concern or Problem

Jacinta has experienced increased anxiety and distress since being asked out by Bruce, which is making it difficult to communicate with him. There had been growing distress before this related to experiences of racism and hate incidents involving her store. **Jacinta recognized that she has not been effectively using her support system, often not offering them the opportunity to support her in aspects of her life.**

Legal and Ethical Issues

Jacinta's husband died in an accident due to unsafe work conditions that were not up to code. Although she received a settlement and moved, people occasionally ask her what happened to her husband, including advocacy groups that monitor the work conditions at the plant where her husband worked.

Theoretical Aspects of the Case Formulation

Jacinta was engaged in the therapy process reflectively and emotionally. Emergent from this, she developed new understandings of her emotional reaction to Bruce. The case formulation reflects her growth in self-awareness, particularly emotional self-awareness, while illustrating how deepening self-awareness is related to the change process.

EXAMPLE CASE FORMULATION FOR JACINTA: THEORETICAL ASPECTS OF THE CASE FORMULATION

Client Strengths and Resources

Jacinta is an intelligent, reflective woman who demonstrated resiliency as a single mother, widow, and business owner. She has a good support system, including family, friends, and community. In addition, she is recognized as a

EXAMPLE CASE FORMULATION FOR JACINTA: THEORETICAL ASPECTS OF THE CASE FORMULATION (*Continued*)

leader in her community for providing space for meetings for groups she is involved with and space for community children to play.

Areas to Follow Up or Clarify

• Jacinta has not been able to identify many things she does for herself, such as hobbies, self-care, and engagement with other interests. Identifying these may be useful for incorporating into self-care and coping strategies.

Biological and Physical Considerations

Jacinta has no known health issues impacting her.

Areas to Follow Up or Clarify

• Jacinta's health anxiety has emerged since her husband's death. At this time, there is no evidence of any active health issues.

Family and Social Considerations

Jacinta is close with her family, including her extended family. She described her family growing up as close. They were poor, with both her parents often working two jobs to make ends meet. She moved away from Albuquerque, which is where her parents and most of her siblings live, after her husband's death. She still visits them several times a year.

Jacinta's oldest son's father is a college boyfriend she has not had contact with since before her son's birth. His parents never knew about the pregnancy. Her ex-boyfriend tried to talk her into getting an abortion and became angry and emotionally abusive when she refused. She met her husband several years later. After they married, he adopted her son, and they had a second son. She described a good marriage, indicating he was a great father. He died 4 years ago in a work accident, leading to her moving to Colorado. She has many aunts, uncles, and cousins in Colorado with whom she has been close since childhood. They continue to be supportive and active in the lives of Jacinta and her children.

Jacinta has a strong support system in her community outside of family, including regular customers at her store, families that attend the meetings at her store, and children who play in a playground behind the store after school. She has increasingly been viewed as a leader in her community. **Over the course of therapy, Jacinta began recognizing that while she has a strong support system, she does not always use it to receive support in some areas of her life.**

(*continues*)

EXAMPLE CASE FORMULATION FOR JACINTA: THEORETICAL ASPECTS OF THE CASE FORMULATION (*Continued*)

Areas to Follow Up or Clarify

- ~~Although Jacinta has a strong support system, it appears she may not be using this for support in some areas of her life, such as grieving for her husband, health anxiety, and worry about her children's safety.~~ **There has been some improvement in Jacinta's use of her support system, but it is still in process.**

School and Employment Considerations

Jacinta owns a successful small business that she enjoys. She experiences stress, worry, and fear from receiving racist messages regarding her business. It is unclear whether these are directed at the business in general or the meetings she hosts in a space in the back of her building. While her business is successful, she has some anxiety about being able to sustain it, **especially if she were to become sick**.

Areas to Follow Up or Clarify

- There are markers suggesting that she is worried about her business, at least partially because it provides security for her children. This is still being clarified with the client.

Cultural Considerations

Jacinta identifies proudly as Latina. **The father of Jacinta's first son is White, and she believes that the primary reason he ended the relationship and pressured her to have an abortion was because she was not White. She believes he was interested in her because she was "exotic" and was never serious about their relationship. Her husband, and the father of her second son, was also Latino. She has not dated since his death, but recently, she was asked out by a White man, which prompted significant anxiety. She has come to recognize that the anxiety was connected to him being White and fears that he may, like the father of her first son, not truly be interested in her because she is Latina. This concern decreased over the course of therapy, and they began dating.**

Jacinta's shop has received numerous racially based hate messages through social media and mailed letters. There have also been a couple of incidences of racist graffiti painted on her store. She is involved with several advocacy groups, primarily focused on the Latinx community and immigrant issues. These groups have provided meaning and community for Jacinta and her family.

EXAMPLE CASE FORMULATION FOR JACINTA: THEORETICAL ASPECTS OF THE CASE FORMULATION (*Continued*)

Areas to Follow Up or Clarify

- ~~Jacinta had a strong reaction to being asked out by a White man who had become a close friend. Some markers suggest that this may be related to his being White; however, this still needs to be clarified.~~

- Jacinta is unclear whether the racially motivated hate incidents are connected to her store selling Latin American and Caribbean products or the groups that she hosts at the store. It is unclear if clarifying this would affect her emotions and/or decisions about her store or these groups.

Systemic Issues

On the occasions Jacinta has called the police about the hate messages and graffiti, she felt the police were dismissive of her and did not take the issue seriously, including questioning her assumption that these were racially motivated. The messages and graffiti include racial slurs and stereotypes, making the racist motivations evident, but the police still questioned it. Jacinta reports feeling less safe due to this, including not being confident that the police will prioritize her safety and that of her family and community. She is angry that the police were not convinced that the messages she received were racially based.

Areas to Follow Up or Clarify

- None at this time.

Self-Awareness and Motivation

Jacinta has good self-awareness in most areas of her life; however, she has recognized some important areas where she lacks clarity. Self-awareness is a priority for her, including serving as a primary motivating force for beginning therapy. Her motivation for therapy is strong. She is engaged in the process, pushes herself, engages in journaling outside of therapy, and prioritizes making it to therapy even when scheduling challenges emerge.

Areas to Follow Up or Clarify

- ~~In the first session, Jacinta showed hesitation about the therapist and her ability to understand her. It is not clear if this impacts her motivation.~~

Here-and-Now

Jacinta can work in the here-and-now intrapersonally and interpersonally; however, there are times when this becomes too intense for her. **Over the course of therapy, this decreased, and she has not felt overwhelmed by this in a couple of months, even when discussing difficult emotions and topics.**

(*continues*)

EXAMPLE CASE FORMULATION FOR JACINTA: THEORETICAL ASPECTS OF THE CASE FORMULATION (*Continued*)

Areas to Follow Up or Clarify

- I will try to clarify better when Jacinta feels overwhelmed in working in the here-and-now to address this feeling of overwhelm. This will also be important in helping follow the client's lead regarding pacing.

Existential Givens

Death and Finiteness

Jacinta reported that her anxiety about her health increased significantly in recent years to the point where she often ruminates about bodily experiences that she worries may be a symptom of a serious illness. In discussing these in therapy, Jacinta recognized that these may be connected to her husband's death, which, in addition to grieving, prompted reflections on her own mortality. **As the health anxiety continued to be explored, an additional connection emerged with fears of dying and leaving her sons without a parent or becoming ill with a serious illness and not being able to take care of her sons.**

Areas to Follow Up or Clarify

- ~~While some of Jacinta's anxiety about health has been clarified, there are markers suggesting that there are other factors contributing to this that are not yet clear.[5]~~

Freedom, Responsibility, and Agency

Although Jacinta is typically good at making decisions, even tough decisions, she described feeling constrained in aspects of her life recently. This includes difficulty with decision making, most notably how to respond to Bruce asking her on a date. **As she has become aware of the pattern of taking on too much responsibility, this has begun to subside, and Jacinta is able to make decisions again more easily.**

Areas to Follow Up or Clarify

- ~~A few markers suggest that Jacinta tends to feel overresponsible in her relationships, which may contribute to feeling constrained. This has not been confirmed with Jacinta.~~

---

[5]This issue has been addressed in this context and can, therefore, be removed; however, the case formulation addresses other possible contributing factors elsewhere.

EXAMPLE CASE FORMULATION FOR JACINTA: THEORETICAL ASPECTS OF THE CASE FORMULATION (*Continued*)

Relationships, Isolation, and Alienation

Jacinta generally has a strong social support system with good family relationships, close friends, and a strong community. **Despite these good relationships, she described a sense of isolation from them that has been clarified over time. In part, this sense of isolation is because she has not shared difficult aspects of her life, such as her grief from losing her husband, with her friends. She has consistently experienced isolation and loneliness since her husband's death. Related to her health concerns are her experiences of existential isolation in imagining what it would be like if she were to get sick. She also experienced existential loneliness, fearing that even her close friends and family cannot understand her situation as a young widow raising two sons.**

Areas to Follow Up or Clarify

- ~~Jacinta's description of relationships suggests feeling a distance from them, even though they are close.~~

- ~~Jacinta does not appear to rely on her support system with aspects of her life, including not sharing certain struggles even with close friends and family.~~

- **We are continuing to explore and better understand Jacinta's emotional reactions in her new relationship with Bruce. She has had some emotional responses on dates that continue to surprise her.**

Emotions and Embodiment

Jacinta is generally open to being with her emotional experiences and talking about them; however, when they reach a certain level of intensity, she tends to "freeze." **It is more difficult to talk about sadness and grief. While she discusses her "worries" with friends and family, there are certain worries, particularly her health worries and worries about her children, that she struggles with sharing.** Jacinta has fear and anxiety about the racial messages directed at her business, including how this may impact her children and possibly other people in her family. In addition to the fear and anxiety, Jacinta is angry about various ways racism has impacted her, including contributing to her husband's death and the hate messages at her store. **Gradually, Jacinta has acknowledged her anger more and discussed it in session. She is beginning to channel her anger into the advocacy groups, helping sustain her motivation to advocate for change.**

Jacinta also has increasing anxiety and ruminations about health concerns, **which have been clarified over time. As she has better understood her health anxiety, she has begun considering who in her family she wants**

(continues)

EXAMPLE CASE FORMULATION FOR JACINTA: THEORETICAL ASPECTS OF THE CASE FORMULATION (*Continued*)

to discuss this with. Her anxiety and ruminations decreased slightly with planning to talk to family members about this.

Areas to Follow Up or Clarify

- ~~There are some emotions that Jacinta has more difficulty talking about. She recognizes this but does not yet understand why.~~

- **Jacinta has recognized that her relationship with her first son's father continues to affect her emotions, including in relationships. We have been focusing on trying to clarify this.**

- ~~Various markers suggest that Jacinta struggles to know what to do with her anger about racism, including how it contributed to her husband's death and the hate messages at her store. She acknowledges the anger but focuses on the fear and anxiety.~~

- ~~Jacinta generally manages her anxiety well but has been struggling with anxiety related to her business and health concerns that are not yet clear.~~

Meaning

Jacinta's central sources of meaning are her children, family, community, and store. She also finds meaning in advocating for the Latinx community and immigrants to the United States. **The meaning connected with the advocacy groups has increased as she has begun channeling her anger and pain into her advocacy.**

Areas to Follow Up or Clarify

- There have been challenges to aspects of Jacinta's meaning with hate messages targeting her store and concern that her involvement with the advocacy groups may be creating safety issues for her family. **She is beginning to use her anger as motivation with the advocacy groups she hosts.**

Daimonic

Jacinta has shown the ability to creatively use strong emotions, channeling them toward good causes, such as her work with the advocacy groups. Some of her involvement with this was inspired by her husband's death, which was caused by unsafe work conditions. **At first, she channeled her sadness, anxiety, and fear; however, more recently, it also included creatively using her anger toward motivation for the advocacy groups.**

Areas to Follow Up or Clarify

- None at this time.

EXAMPLE CASE FORMULATION FOR JACINTA: THEORETICAL ASPECTS OF THE CASE FORMULATION (*Continued*)

Self-Acceptance

Jacinta can be critical of herself as a mother; she particularly worries whether some of her involvements, such as advocacy groups, may put her children at risk. She has also been critical of herself regarding her relationship with Daniel's father. However, Jacinta typically can accept herself, including mistakes and flaws.

Areas to Follow Up or Clarify

- None at this time.

Client–Therapist Relationship

Jacinta shows signs of a strong therapy relationship overall. In the first session, there were brief concerns about whether I would be able to understand aspects of her life and experience. In earlier sessions, she **was also** overwhelmed by emotion in response to my presence and empathy. **This has subsided.**

Areas to Follow Up or Clarify

- ~~Jacinta voiced concern in the first session about whether I would be able to understand aspects of her life and experience.~~[6]

- ~~Jacinta worried, at times, about causing me to feel bad, which appears to have contributed to hesitancy in sharing intense emotions.~~

- ~~Jacinta has occasionally been overwhelmed by the experience of my presence and empathy. At first, she struggled to tell me this because she did not want to be critical of me.~~

- **While the areas where Jacinta held back in the therapy relationship out of concern for me have been addressed, I will watch for the possibility of this returning in the future.**

Therapist's Perspective on the Client–Therapist Relationship

The therapy relationship from early on has been strong despite some periods of hesitancy. It does not appear these were from Jacinta not trusting me; instead, they appeared connected to common patterns in her life of focusing on the needs of others first and trying to be considerate. **In addition, she has sometimes struggled to set boundaries with people she feels have good intentions. This contributed to her hesitating to ask me to slow down or back off when she was feeling overwhelmed.**

---

[6]The areas to follow up or clarify have gradually been modified and replaced over the course of therapy as the client–therapist relationship has evolved, culminating in the fourth bullet point as the one area that needs attention as of Session 30.

Treatment Planning

Jacinta's engagement in the therapy process and growing self-awareness led to important changes in the goals. This is similar to Hank's situation; however, Hank and Jacinta were different in the process of gaining awareness that informed changes to the goals. While Hank had strong protections that limited his awareness, Jacinta was more openly engaged. Therefore, even when similar therapy strategies were employed (vivification, searching strategies), they often looked different, as illustrated in some of the sample dialogues from the therapy overview.

EXAMPLE CASE FORMULATION FOR JACINTA: TREATMENT PLANNING

Narrative of the Client's Desired Outcome

Jacinta is striving for a future centered on her children, family, and local community. She hopes her shop continues to thrive and be viewed as a center-piece of the local community, especially for the Latinx and other minoritized communities. **While she would like the hate messages to stop, she knows that is beyond her control and would like her community to take a stronger stand together against such incidents, including advocating for the police to take the hate messages more seriously. She is beginning to channel her anger into stronger encouragement for her community to take action.** Jacinta would like to remarry someone who is also invested in their local community. She would like her concerns about her health to decrease. In general, she wants to be more confident in her decisions and how she is living her life.

Areas to Follow Up or Clarify

- Further clarification on Jacinta's desire to remarry may be helpful, including clarifying what she is looking for in a relationship.

Initial Client Goals

- deepen her self-awareness about her emotional reactions in the context of potential dating relationships, including her reaction to being asked out on a date by Bruce

- better understand her emotions

- decrease her "worry" about her children and her store

- decrease her health concerns and related rumination patterns

EXAMPLE CASE FORMULATION FOR JACINTA: TREATMENT PLANNING (*Continued*)

Emergent Client Goals

- facilitate grieving for her husband
- become more comfortable being vulnerable about her children and health concerns with close friends and family
- improve her ability to use her anger in constructive ways

Anticipated Challenges and/or Barriers

Jacinta is a single mother with significant responsibilities and related stress, including financial limitations. The hate messages her store receives are beyond her control and likely will continue causing stress.

Areas to Follow Up or Clarify

- Jacinta has struggled, at times, in being vulnerable with the therapist, and it appears this may be occurring with other relationships, limiting her ability to take full advantage of her support systems. **This has been improving in recent weeks.**

Existential–Humanistic Treatment Strategies and Interventions

- presence to facilitate self-exploration and relational depth in therapy; ~~however, it will be important to be cautious with this and watch for signs that this may feel overwhelming or intrusive~~[7]

- empathy and the facilitation of emotional processing to promote self-acceptance and emotional exploration, including grief, anxiety, and anger. ~~However, it will be important to gradually incorporate empathy more and be cautious to decrease the likelihood of contributing to feeling emotionally or interpersonally overwhelmed.~~

- searching strategies to promote self-awareness

- vivification of protections to promote self-awareness and agency

- here-and-now interventions for deepening trust in the therapy relationships and promoting intrapersonal and interpersonal self-awareness. **This can also serve as a model for changing her communication patterns with family and friends to deepen these relationships.**

(continues)

---

[7]The latter half of the first two strategies or interventions were addressed over time, so the second half of each sentence can now be removed.

EXAMPLE CASE FORMULATION FOR JACINTA: TREATMENT PLANNING (*Continued*)

- here-and-now interventions focusing on helping Jacinta find creative ways to use her anger

- self-disclosure to build the therapy alliance and model ways to approach relationships and emotions

Integrative Strategies

- journaling with some creative arts strategies integrated to facilitate emotional processing and self-awareness
- journaling focused on finding creative ways to use her anger
- mindfulness strategies to promote self-awareness and acceptance of emotions
- breathing strategies for self-care and emotional regulation

Treatment Progress

Jacinta has made significant progress with self-awareness, which was her primary goal when entering therapy. In addition to understanding her reaction to Bruce asking her out, she has deepened her self-awareness in various areas, including her grief for her husband; emotions connected to Greg, her former boyfriend; anger about experiences of racism; and her worry and anxiety about her health concerns. Her anxieties have decreased in all areas, and she feels more comfortable with the anxiety she continues to experience. She is able to listen to her emotions better and make sense of them. Jacinta began being more vulnerable in several close relationships. With Bruce, she has taken the risk to begin a dating relationship. When she has strong emotions come up with Bruce, she no longer retreats from the relationship and, instead, seeks to understand the emotion. Bruce is one of the relationships in which she is also beginning to be more vulnerable. Jacinta is less afraid of her anger and more able to embrace and creatively use it.

Epilogue

Concluding Thoughts on Existential–Humanistic Therapy Case Formulation

Existential–humanistic (EH) case formulation fills several critical gaps for EH therapy. First, it provides a model for guiding EH therapists with a basic structure while maintaining the flexibility and fluidity essential to EH therapy. Second, this approach is deeply client centered, which few approaches to case formulation have been able to achieve. An exception is Goldman and Greenberg's (2015) *Emotion-Focused Therapy Case Formulation*, which is also client centered. Third, this provides a guide to learning and evaluating EH case formulations. This is particularly useful for students, supervisors, and professors learning, teaching, and evaluating case formulations in graduate programs and training sites. Fourth, this case formulation model provides a foundation for demonstrating that EH therapy is being practiced consistent with evidence-based practice in psychology. Fifth, this provides a structure that can inform existential–integrative approaches to therapy. Last, this provides a basic structure for researchers to conduct outcome studies on EH therapy. We hope this will increase the research on EH therapy and its components.

Each section of the case formulation has been discussed in detail, along with an example, Rasheeda. The example of Rasheeda is more detailed and provides some insight into the EH therapy process. The second two examples in Chapter 9 are briefer, focusing more specifically on the case formulation. The varied examples provide greater clarity pertaining to how the different sections can be developed with specific clients.

https://doi.org/10.1037/0000464-011
Case Formulation in Existential–Humanistic Therapy, by L. Hoffman and H. P. Cleare-Hoffman

FUTURE DIRECTIONS

We have structured this approach to EH case formulation to be adaptable. It can be completed in different ways. We recommend that the main sections be written in paragraph form with bullet points for the Areas to Follow Up or Clarify. This allows for an easy transition into a report, when needed, by deleting the bullet points. Using bullet points for areas to follow up or clarify can be useful when using the case formulation to enhance and guide EH therapy. The therapist can use this to track emerging markers, themes, and patterns that are not yet clear and/or confirmed with the client. We hope practitioners and scholars will work with this initial framework to develop adaptations stylized to their unique styles and different therapeutic contexts.

The Evidence-Based Foundations of Existential–Humanistic Therapy (Hoffman & Lac, 2025) is intended as a companion volume to this book. While the companion volume demonstrates that there is already strong research support for EH therapy, we hope that this case formulation model can be used as a basic structure for outcome research on EH psychotherapy. A primary limitation of outcome research to date has been the lack of a structure that can be used to guide EH therapy. The publication of *Case Formulation in Existential–Humanistic Therapy* opens new possibilities for research. We hope to see many dissertations and grants funding research that will build on this foundation in the coming years.

CONCLUSION

EH therapy is a unique approach to psychotherapy that, according to Wampold (2008), provides an ideal foundation for psychotherapy. The principles and stances of EH therapy have been strongly supported by the research literature (see Hoffman & Lac, 2025; Wampold, 2008). The framework discussed in this book allows for various other approaches to be integrated as beneficial to the client. The EH case formulation approach is designed to aid therapists in better "seeing" their clients holistically and developing a relational depth that is healing to clients and facilitates sustained changes.

Existential–Humanistic Case Formulation

Client name: Report date:

Client age: Gender identification and pronouns:

Therapist: Supervisor:

Number of sessions: Frequency of sessions:

BRIEF HOLISTIC CLIENT NARRATIVE (3–5 PARAGRAPHS)

CONCERN OR PROBLEM IDENTIFICATION

Client's Description of the Concern or Problem

Initial Client Perspective on the Concern or Problem

Emergent Client Perspective on the Concern or Problem

Areas to Follow Up or Clarify

Diagnosis of Systems or Contextual Issues Impacting Psychological Health

Implications of the Concern or Problem

Legal and Ethical Issues

ICD-11 Diagnosis or *DSM-5* Diagnosis (if required or beneficial; if beneficial to understanding the client's challenges, add contextualization of the diagnosis)

Alternative Diagnosis (e.g., Psychodynamic Diagnostic Manual 2; Power Threat Meaning Framework; recovery-orientated narrative; Pavlo et al., 2019)

THEORETICAL ASPECTS OF THE CASE FORMULATION

Client Strengths and Resources

Areas to Follow Up or Clarify

Biological and Physical Considerations

Areas to Follow Up or Clarify

Family and Social Considerations

Areas to Follow Up or Clarify

School and Employment Considerations

Areas to Follow Up or Clarify

Cultural Considerations

Areas to Follow Up or Clarify

Systemic Issues

Areas to Follow Up or Clarify

Self-Awareness and Motivation

Areas to Follow Up or Clarify

Here-and-Now

Areas to Follow Up or Clarify

Existential Givens

Death and Finiteness

Areas to follow up or clarify

Freedom, Responsibility, and Agency

Areas to follow up or clarify

Relationships, Isolation, and Alienation

Areas to follow up or clarify

Emotions and Embodiment

Areas to follow up or clarify

Meaning

Areas to Follow Up or Clarify

Daimonic

Areas to Follow Up or Clarify

Self-Acceptance

Areas to Follow Up or Clarify

Client–Therapist Relationship

Areas to Follow Up or Clarify

Therapist's Perspective on the Client–Therapist Relationship

TREATMENT PLANNING

Narrative of the Client's Desired Outcome

Areas to Follow Up or Clarify

Initial Client Goals

Emergent Client Goals

Treatment Goals (optional)

Anticipated Challenges and/or Barriers

Areas to Follow Up or Clarify

Existential–Humanistic Treatment Strategies and Interventions

Integrative Strategies

Treatment Progress (initially left blank)

Support for Treatment Approaches, Stances, and/or Techniques (optional)

ADDITIONAL INFORMATION

Recommended Reading for Existential–Humanistic Theory and Psychotherapy

This appendix is divided into three sections: (a) theory recommendations, (b) intervention recommendations, and (c) using research to support existential–humanistic psychotherapy.

THEORY RECOMMENDATIONS

Diagnostic Alternatives

Karter, J., & Kamens, S. (2019). Toward conceptual competence in psychiatric diagnosis: An ecological model for critiques of the *DSM*. In S. Steingard (Ed.), *Critical psychiatry: Controversies and clinical implications* (pp. 17–69). Springer. https://doi.org/10.1007/978-3-030-02732-2_2

Pavlo, A. J. (2026). A little "stand-offish": Existential and humanistic diagnostic perspectives on diagnosis. In L. Hoffman (Ed.), *APA handbook of humanistic and existential psychology* (Vol. 1, pp. 349–364). American Psychological Association. https://doi.org/10.1037/0000431-015

Cultural and Systemic Considerations

Hoffman, L., Cleare-Hoffman, H. P., Granger, N., Jr., & St. John, D. (Eds.). (2020). *Humanistic approaches to multiculturalism and diversity: Perspectives on existence and difference.* Routledge. https://doi.org/10.4324/9781351133357

Hoffman, L., Cleare-Hoffman, H. P., & Jackson, T. (2014). Humanistic psychology and multiculturalism: History, current status, and advancements. In K. J. Schneider, J. F. Pierson, & J. F. T. Bugental (Eds.), *The handbook of humanistic psychology: Theory, research, and practice* (2nd ed., pp. 41–55). Sage. https://doi.org/10.4135/9781483387864.n4

Lorenz, H., & James, S. (2026). Liberation psychologies and decolonialities: Defecting from environments of domination to build spaces of collective agency, prefigurative politics, and ecological justice. In L. Hoffman (Ed.), *APA handbook of humanistic and existential psychology* (Vol. 1, pp. 647–668). American Psychological Association. https://doi.org/10.1037/0000431-028

Newton, M. B., & Jackson, T. R. (2026). Integrating multicultural perspectives. In L. Hoffman (Ed.), *APA handbook of humanistic and existential psychology* (Vol. 2, pp. 31–48). American Psychological Association. https://doi.org/10.1037/0000432-002

Self-Awareness

Spaeth, D., Vanderhoff, J. A., Pintauro, M., & Hoffman, L. (2025). Authenticity, self-awareness, and facing life directly in existential–humanistic psychotherapy. In L. Hoffman & V. Lac (Eds.), *The evidence-based foundations of existential–humanistic therapy* (pp. 183–206). American Psychological Association. https://doi.org/10.1037/0000446-008

Here-and-Now

Bugental, J. F. T. (1999). *Psychotherapy isn't what you think.* Zeig, Tucker & Co.
Underwood, J. J. (2025). Here-and-now work in existential–humanistic psychotherapy. In L. Hoffman & V. Lac (Eds.), *The evidence-based foundations of existential–humanistic therapy* (pp. 207–224). American Psychological Association. https://doi.org/10.1037/0000446-009

Death and Limitations

Becker, E. (1973). *The denial of death.* Free Press.
Pyszczynski, T., & Diarra, M. (2026). Terror management theory: Toward a merger of existential and experimental approaches to understanding human behavior and experience. In L. Hoffman (Ed.), *APA handbook of humanistic and existential psychology* (Vol. 1, pp. 405–430). American Psychological Association. https://doi.org/10.1037/0000431-017
Yalom, I. D. (1980). *Existential psychotherapy.* Basic Books.

Freedom, Responsibility, and Agency

May, R. (1981). *Freedom and destiny.* Norton.
van Deurzen, E. (2026). Contemporary considerations of freedom. In L. Hoffman (Ed.), *APA handbook of humanistic and existential psychology* (Vol. 1, pp. 431–448). American Psychological Association. https://doi.org/10.1037/0000431-018
van Deurzen, E. (in press). *The art of existential freedom: Guide to a wiser life.* Penguin.
Yalom, I. D. (1980). *Existential psychotherapy.* Basic Books.

Relationship, Isolation, and Alienation

Bugental, J. F. T. (1987). *The art of the psychotherapist.* Norton.
Hoffman, L., & Islam, S. (2026). Relationality, isolation, and alienation. In L. Hoffman (Ed.), *APA handbook of humanistic and existential psychology* (Vol. 1, pp. 495–520). American Psychological Association. https://doi.org/10.1037/0000431-021
Mearns, D., & Cooper, M. (2017). *Working at relational depth in counseling and psychotherapy* (2nd ed.). Sage.
Morrill, Z. (2025). Genuineness and the real relationship in existential–humanistic psychotherapy. In L. Hoffman & V. Lac (Eds.), *The evidence-based foundations of existential–humanistic therapy* (pp. 267–292). American Psychological Association. https://doi.org/10.1037/0000446-012
Yalom, I. D. (1980). *Existential psychotherapy.* Basic Books.

Embodiment and Emotions

Bugental, J. F. T. (1987). *The art of the psychotherapist.* Norton.
LeBeau, C. S., Lowe, A. B., & McDonald, H. (2026). Existential anxiety and guilt. In L. Hoffman (Ed.), *APA handbook of humanistic and existential psychology* (Vol. 1, pp. 303–324). American Psychological Association. https://doi.org/10.1037/0000431-013

Varisco, B., & Hoffman, L. (2025). Working with emotions in existential–humanistic psychotherapy. In L. Hoffman & V. Lac (Eds.), *The evidence-based foundations of existential–humanistic therapy* (pp. 157–182). American Psychological Association. https://doi.org/10.1037/0000446-007

Meaning

Frankl, V. (1984). *Man's search for meaning*. Simon & Schuster.

Russo-Netzer, P., & Vos, J. (2026). Meaning interventions: Working with meaning in life in psychological therapies. In L. Hoffman (Ed.), *APA handbook of humanistic and existential psychology* (Vol. 2, pp. 175–206). American Psychological Association. https://doi.org/10.1037/0000432-009

Vos, J. (2025). Working with meaning in life in existential–humanistic psychotherapy. In L. Hoffman & V. Lac (Eds.), *The evidence-based foundations of existential–humanistic therapy* (pp. 225–252). American Psychological Association. https://doi.org/10.1037/0000446-010

Vos, J. (2026). Meaning in life and society. In L. Hoffman (Ed.), *APA handbook of humanistic and existential psychology* (Vol. 2, pp. 501–534). American Psychological Association. https://doi.org/10.1037/0000432-025

Yalom, I. D. (1980). *Existential psychotherapy*. Basic Books.

Daimonic

Diamond, S. A. (1996). *Anger, madness, and the daimonic*. State University of New York Press.

Diamond, S. A. (2026). The psychology and psychotherapy of evil: Encountering the daimonic. In L. Hoffman (Ed.), *APA handbook of humanistic and existential psychology* (Vol. 1, pp. 365–404). American Psychological Association. https://doi.org/10.1037/0000431-016

May, R. (1969). *Love and will*. Delta.

Sense of Self and Self-Acceptance

Bland, A. M. (2026). Self-actualization and coactualization. In L. Hoffman (Ed.), *APA handbook of humanistic and existential psychology* (Vol. 1, pp. 325–348). American Psychological Association. https://doi.org/10.1037/0000431-014

Hanna, F. J., & Givens, J. (2026). The existential–phenomenological self: Perspectives and insights. In L. Hoffman (Ed.), *APA handbook of humanistic and existential psychology* (Vol. 1, pp. 283–302). American Psychological Association. https://doi.org/10.1037/0000431-012

Hoffman, L., Lopez, A., & Moats, M. (2013). Humanistic psychology and self-acceptance. In M. Bernard (Ed.), *The strength of self-acceptance: Theory, research, and practice* (pp. 3–17). Springer. https://doi.org/10.1007/978-1-4614-6806-6_1

Hsu, A. Y. J. (2025). The self in existential–humanistic psychotherapy. In L. Hoffman & V. Lac (Eds.), *The evidence-based foundations of existential–humanistic therapy* (pp. 311–332). American Psychological Association. https://doi.org/10.1037/0000446-014

TREATMENT INTERVENTIONS

Treatment Interventions

Christensen, R., & Vincent, A. (2025). Understanding acceptance in existential–humanistic psychotherapy. In L. Hoffman & V. Lac (Eds.), *The evidence-based foundations of existential–humanistic therapy* (pp. 253–266). American Psychological Association. https://doi.org/10.1037/0000446-011

Krug, O. T. (2019). Existential-humanistic and existential-integrative therapy: Method and practice. In E. van Durzen, E. Craig, A. Längle, K. J. Schneider, D. Tantam, & S. du Pluck (Eds.), *The Wiley world handbook of existential therapy*. Wiley.

Krug, O. T., Bradshaw, C., Ratner, J., & Sánchez-Mazarro, A. (2025). Therapeutic presence in existential–humanistic psychotherapy. In L. Hoffman & V. Lac (Eds.), *The evidence-based foundations of existential–humanistic therapy* (pp. 103–130). American Psychological Association. https://doi.org/10.1037/0000446-005

Schneider, K. J., & Krug, O. T. (2017). *Existential–humanistic therapy* (2nd ed.). American Psychological Association. https://doi.org/10.1037/0000042-000

Sebree, D., Jr., & Brown, V. (2025). Therapist self-disclosure in existential–humanistic psychotherapy. In L. Hoffman & V. Lac (Eds.), *The evidence-based foundations of existential–humanistic therapy* (pp. 293–310). American Psychological Association. https://doi.org/10.1037/0000446-013

Spaeth, D. (2026). Foundations of humanistic and existential therapy. In L. Hoffman (Ed.), *APA handbook of humanistic and existential psychology* (Vol. 2, pp. 3–30). American Psychological Association. https://doi.org/10.1037/0000432-001

Vanhooren, S., & Schneider, K. J. (2026). Humanistic and existential therapies: An integrative perspective. In L. Hoffman (Ed.), *APA handbook of humanistic and existential psychology* (Vol. 2, pp. 351–368). American Psychological Association. https://doi.org/10.1037/0000432-018

Presence

Geller, S. M., & Greenberg, L. S. (2022). *Therapeutic presence: A mindful approach to effective therapeutic relationships* (2nd ed.). American Psychological Association. https://doi.org/10.1037/0000315-000

Krug, O. T. (2009). James Bugental and Irvin Yalom: Two masters of existential therapy cultivate presence in the therapeutic encounter. *Journal of Humanistic Psychology, 49*(3), 329–354. https://doi.org/10.1177/0022167809334001

Krug, O. T., Bradshaw, C., Ratner, J., & Sánchez-Mazarro, A. (2025). Therapeutic presence inexistential–humanistic psychotherapy. In L. Hoffman & V. Lac (Eds.), *The evidence-based foundations of existential–humanistic therapy* (pp. 103–130). American Psychological Association. https://doi.org/10.1037/0000446-005

Schneider, K. J. (2015). Presence: The core contextual factor of effective psychotherapy. *Existential Analysis, 2*(2), 304–312.

Empathy

Bohart, A. C., & Greenberg, L. S. (Eds.). (1997). *Empathy reconsidered: New directions in psychotherapy*. American Psychological Association. https://doi.org/10.1037/10226-000

Bohart, A. C., Shapiro, J. L., & Byock, G. (2025). Empathy in existential–humanistic psychotherapy. In L. Hoffman & V. Lac (Eds.), *The evidence-based foundations of existential–humanistic therapy* (pp. 131–156). American Psychological Association. https://doi.org/10.1037/0000446-006

Hoffman, L. (2020). Culture and empathy in humanistic psychology. In L. Hoffman, H. P. Cleare-Hoffman, N. Granger, Jr., & D. St. John (Eds.), *Humanistic approaches to multiculturalism and diversity: Perspectives on existence and difference* (pp. 103–116). Routledge. https://doi.org/10.4324/9781351133357-9

Genuineness and the Real Relationship

Gelso, C. J. (2010). *The real relationship in psychotherapy: The hidden foundation of change*. American Psychological Association. https://doi.org/10.1037/12349-000

Morrill, Z. (2025). Genuineness and the real relationship in existential–humanistic psychotherapy. In L. Hoffman & V. Lac (Eds.), *The evidence-based foundations of existential–humanistic therapy* (pp. 267–292). American Psychological Association. https://doi.org/10.1037/0000446-012

Rogers, C. R. (1951). *Client-centered therapy*. Houghton Mifflin.

Working With Emotions, Embodiment, and What Is Present

See Emotions and Embodiment under Theory Recommendations.

Understanding and Working With Protections and Resistance

Bugental, J. F. T. (1999). *Psychotherapy isn't what you think*. Zeig, Tucker & Co.

Schneider, K. J., & Krug, O. T. (2017). *Existential–humanistic therapy* (2nd ed.). American Psychological Association. https://doi.org/10.1037/0000042-000

Meaning-Centered Interventions

See meaning under Theory Recommendations.

Authenticity, Self-Awareness, and Facing Life Directly

Bugental, J. F. T. (1965). *The search for authenticity*. Holt, Rinehart & Winston.

Spaeth, D., Vanderhoff, J. A., Pintauro, M., & Hoffman, L. (2025). Authenticity, self-awareness, and facing life directly in existential–humanistic psychotherapy. In L. Hoffman & V. Lac (Eds.), *The evidence-based foundations of existential–humanistic therapy* (pp. 183–206). American Psychological Association. https://doi.org/10.1037/0000446-008

Wang, X. (2019). The symbol of the iron house: From survivalism to existentialism. In L. Hoffman, M. Yang, M. Mansilla, J. Dias, M. Moats, & T. Claypool (Eds.), *Existential psychology East-West* (Vol. 2, pp. 3–16). University Professors Press.

Here-and-Now

See Here-and-Now under Theory Recommendations.

Positive Regard and Acceptance

Christensen, R., & Vincent, A. (2025). Understanding acceptance in existential–humanistic psychotherapy. In L. Hoffman & V. Lac (Eds.), *The evidence-based foundations of existential–humanistic therapy* (pp. 253–266). American Psychological Association. https://doi.org/10.1037/0000446-011

Rogers, C. R. (1951). *Client-centered therapy*. Houghton Mifflin.

Self-Disclosure

Farber, B. A. (2006). *Self-disclosure in psychotherapy*. Guilford Press.

Sebree, D., Jr., & Brown, V. (2025). Therapist self-disclosure in existential–humanistic psychotherapy. In L. Hoffman & V. Lac (Eds.), *The evidence-based foundations of existential–humanistic therapy* (pp. 293–310). American Psychological Association. https://doi.org/10.1037/0000446-013

Integrative Strategies

Schneider, K. J. (2007). *Existential-integrative psychotherapy: Guideposts to the core of practice.* Routledge.

Vanhooren, S., & Schneider, K. J. (2026). Humanistic and existential therapies: An integrative perspective. In L. Hoffman (Ed.), *APA handbook of humanistic and existential psychology* (Vol. 2, pp. 351–368). American Psychological Association. https://doi.org/10.1037/0000432-018

Experiential Techniques

Creative and Expressive Arts Interventions

Herron, S. A. (2026). Expressive arts therapy. In L. Hoffman (Ed.), *APA handbook of humanistic and existential psychology* (Vol. 2, pp. 153–174). American Psychological Association. https://doi.org/10.1037/0000432-008

Serlin, I. A., Ho, R. T. H., Kurter Musnitsky, F., & Kennedy, J. R. (2025). The creative and expressive arts therapies and existential–humanistic psychotherapy. In L. Hoffman & V. Lac (Eds.), *The evidence-based foundations of existential–humanistic therapy* (pp. 359–380). American Psychological Association. https://doi.org/10.1037/0000446-016

Mindfulness

Rockwell, D., Johnson, O. O., & Scharding, S. (2025). Integrative considerations of mindfulness in existential–humanistic psychotherapy. In L. Hoffman & V. Lac (Eds.), *The evidence-based foundations of existential–humanistic therapy* (pp. 335–357). American Psychological Association. https://doi.org/10.1037/0000446-015

USING RESEARCH TO SUPPORT EXISTENTIAL–HUMANISTIC PSYCHOTHERAPY

Hoffman, L. (2024). The possibilities and slippery slope of evidence-based practice in psychology: Why humanistic and existential psychologists must engage the conversation. *The Humanistic Psychologist, 52*(3), 318–324. https://doi.org/10.1037/hum0000347

Hoffman, L. (2025). Approaching existential–humanistic psychotherapy from an evidence-based perspective. In L. Hoffman & V. Lac (Eds.), *The evidence-based foundations of existential–humanistic therapy* (pp. 11–38). American Psychological Association. https://doi.org/10.1037/0000446-002

Hoffman, L., & Lac, V. (Eds.). (2025). *The evidence-based foundations of existential–humanistic therapy.* American Psychological Association. https://doi.org/10.1037/0000446-000

Zegers, H., & Vanhooren, S. (2026). The use of research in humanistic and existential psychotherapy. In L. Hoffman (Ed.), *APA handbook of humanistic and existential psychology* (Vol. 2, pp. 133–152). American Psychological Association. https://doi.org/10.1037/0000432-007

REFERENCES

Addis, M. E., & Cardemil, E. V. (2006). Does manualization improve therapy outcomes? In J. C. Norcross, L. E. Beutler, & R. L. Levant (Eds.), *Evidence-based practices in mental health: Debate and dialogue on the fundamental questions* (pp. 131–160). American Psychological Association. https://doi.org/10.1037/11265-003

American Psychiatric Association. (2022). *Diagnostic and statistical manual of mental disorders* (5th ed., text rev.). https://doi.org/10.1176/appi.books.9780890425596

American Psychological Association. (n.d.-a). Agency. In *APA dictionary of psychology*. Retrieved April 20, 2024, from https://dictionary.apa.org/agency

American Psychological Association. (n.d.-b). Culture. In *APA dictionary of psychology*. Retrieved April 20, 2024, from https://dictionary.apa.org/culture

American Psychological Association, Presidential Task Force on Evidence-Based Practice. (2006). Evidence-based practice in psychology. *American Psychologist*, *61*(4), 271–285. https://doi.org/10.1037/0003-066X.61.4.271

Baldwin, J. (1962). *The fire next time*. Vintage.

Barkham, M., & Lambert, M. J. (2021). The efficacy and effectiveness of psychological therapies. In M. Barkham, W. Lutz, & L. G. Castonguay (Eds.), *Bergin and Garfield's handbook of psychotherapy and behavioral change* (50th anniv. ed., pp. 135–189). Wiley.

Beauvoir, S. de. (1976). *The ethics of ambiguity*. Kensington Publishing. (Original work published 1948)

Beauvoir, S. de. (2009). *The second sex* (C. Borde & S. Malovany-Chevallier, Trans.). Alfred A. Knopf. (Original work published 1949)

Becker, E. (1973). *The denial of death*. Free Press.

Becker, E. (1975). *Escape from evil*. Free Press.

Bland, A. M. (2026). Self-actualization and coactualization. In L. Hoffman (Ed.), *APA handbook of humanistic and existential psychology* (Vol. 1, pp. 325–348). American Psychological Association. https://doi.org/10.1037/0000431-014

Bohart, A. C., & Greenberg, L. S. (1997a). Empathy and psychotherapy: An introductory overview. In A. C. Bohart & L. S. Greenberg (Eds.), *Empathy reconsidered: New directions in psychotherapy* (pp. 3–31). American Psychological Association. https://doi.org/10.1037/10226-018

Bohart, A. C., & Greenberg, L. S. (Eds.). (1997b). *Empathy reconsidered: New directions in psychotherapy*. American Psychological Association. https://doi.org/10.1037/10226-000

Bohart, A. C., & Tallman, K. (1999). *How clients make therapy work: The process of active self-healing*. American Psychological Association. https://doi.org/10.1037/10323-000

Bugental, J. F. T. (1965). *The search for authenticity*. Holt, Rinehart & Winston.

Bugental, J. F. T. (1987). *The art of the psychotherapist*. Norton.

Bugental, J. F. T. (1999). *Psychotherapy isn't what you think*. Zeig, Tucker & Co.

Bugental, J. F. T., & Sterling, M. M. (1995). Existential-humanistic psychotherapy: New perspectives. In A. S. Gurman & S. B. Messer (Eds.), *Essential psychotherapies: Theory and practice* (pp. 226–260). Guilford Press.

Camus, A. (1988). *The stranger* (M. Ward, Trans.). Vintage. (Original work published 1942)

Cleare-Hoffman, H. P. (2019). Junkanoo: A Bahamian cultural myth. In L. Hoffman, M. Yang, F. J. Kaklauskas, A. Chan, & M. Mansilla (Eds.), *Existential psychology East-West* (Rev. & expanded ed., Vol. 1, pp. 381–390). University Professors Press.

Cleare-Hoffman, H. P., & Hoffman, L. (2017, August 3–6). *Key influences on the development of existential-humanistic therapy practice* [Poster presentation]. American Psychological Association 125th Annual Conference, Washington, DC, United States.

Cleare-Hoffman, H. P., & Hoffman, L. (2018, August 9–12). Multicultural considerations in existential-humanistic case conceptualization and treatment planning. In L. Hoffman (Chair), *Existential–humanistic case conceptualization and treatment planning* [Symposium]. American Psychological Association 126th Annual Conference, San Francisco, CA, United States.

Cleare-Hoffman, H. P., Hoffman, L., & Paige, J. (2020). Cultural myths, rituals, and festivals. In L. Hoffman, H. P. Cleare-Hoffman, N. Granger, Jr., & D. St. John (Eds.), *Humanistic approaches to multiculturalism and diversity: Perspectives on existence and difference* (pp. 117–127). Routledge. https://doi.org/10.4324/9781351133357-10

Cleary, S. (2022). *How to be authentic: Simone de Beauvoir and the quest for fulfillment*. St. Martin's Essentials.

Cole, T. (2025). Experiential techniques in existential–humanistic psychotherapy. In L. Hoffman & V. Lac (Eds.), *The evidence-based foundations of existential-humanistic therapy* (pp. 381–396). American Psychological Association. https://doi.org/10.1037/0000446-017

Cooper, M., & Law, D. (Eds.). (2018). *Working with goals in psychotherapy and counseling*. Oxford University Press. https://doi.org/10.1093/med-psych/9780198793687.001.0001

Diamond, S. A. (1996). *Anger, madness, and the daimonic: The psychological genesis of violence, evil, and creativity*. State University of New York Press.

Diamond, S. A. (2026). The psychology and psychotherapy of evil: Encountering the daimonic. In L. Hoffman (Ed.), *APA handbook of humanistic and existential psychology* (Vol. 1, pp. 365–404). American Psychological Association. https://doi.org/10.1037/0000431-016

DuBose, T. (2026). Authenticity and genuineness. In L. Hoffman (Ed.), *APA handbook of humanistic and existential psychology* (Vol. 1, pp. 545–564). American Psychological Association. https://doi.org/10.1037/0000431-023

Eells, T. D. (2015). *Psychotherapy case formulation*. American Psychological Association. https://doi.org/10.1037/14667-000

Elkins, D. N. (2009). *Humanistic psychology: A clinical manifesto*. University of the Rockies Press.

Ellenberger, H. F. (1958). A clinical introduction to psychiatric phenomenology and existential analysis. In R. May, E. Angel, & H. F. Ellenberger (Eds.), *Existence: A new dimension in psychiatry and psychology* (pp. 92–124). Jason Aronson.

Falk, J., & Hoffman, L. (Eds.). (2022). *Becoming an existential-humanistic therapist: Narratives from the journey*. University Professors Press.

Fanon, F. (1965). *A dying colonialism* (H. Chevalier, Trans.). Grove Press. (Original work published 1959)

Fanon, F. (2004). *The wretched of the earth* (R. Philcox, Trans.). Grove Press. (Original work published 1963)

Fanon, F. (2008). *Black skin, white masks* (R. Philcox, Trans.). Grove Press. (Original work published 1952)

Feinstein, D., & Krippner, S. (2009). *Personal mythology: Using ritual, dreams, and imagination to discover your inner story* (3rd ed.). Energy Psychology Press.

Frankl, V. E. (1984). *Man's search for meaning*. Simon & Schuster. (Original work published 1946)

Frankl, V. E. (2001). *Yes to life: In spite of everything*. Beacon.

Freire, P. (2009). *Pedagogy of the oppressed* (30th anniv. ed.). Continuum. (Original work published 1970)

Fromm, E. (1941). *Escape from freedom*. Holt.

Geller, S. M., Greenberg, L. S., & Watson, J. C. (2010). Therapist and client perceptions of therapeutic presence: The development of a measure. *Psychotherapy Research, 20*(5), 599–610. https://doi.org/10.1080/10503307.2010.495957

Gelso, C. J., & Silberberg, A. (2016). Strengthening the real relationship: What is a psychotherapist to do? *Practice Innovations, 1*(3), 154–163. https://doi.org/10.1037/pri0000024

Goldman, R. N., & Greenberg, L. S. (2015). *Case formulation in emotion-focused therapy: Co-creating clinical maps for change*. American Psychological Association. https://doi.org/10.1037/14523-000

Greening, T. (1992). Existential challenges and responses. *The Humanistic Psychologist, 20*(1), 111–115. https://doi.org/10.1080/08873267.1992.9986784

Greening, T. (2017). *Words against the void: Poems by an existential psychologist* (Rev. & expanded ed.). University Professors Press.

Hayes, S. C., Strosahl, K. D., & Wilson, K. G. (2016). *Acceptance and commitment therapy: The process and practice of mindful change* (2nd ed.). Guilford Press.

Henretty, J. R., Currier, J. M., Berman, J. S., & Levitt, H. M. (2014). The impact of counselor self-disclosure on clients: A meta-analytic review of experimental and quasi-experimental research. *Journal of Counseling Psychology, 61*(2), 191–207. https://doi.org/10.1037/a0036189

Hill, C. E., Knox, S., & Pinto-Coelho, K. G. (2018). Therapist self-disclosure and immediacy: A qualitative meta-analysis. *Psychotherapy, 55*(4), 445–460. https://doi.org/10.1037/pst0000182

Hocoy, D. (1999). Marginalization among Blacks in South Africa. In J. C. Lasry, J. Adiar, & K. Dion (Eds.), *Latest contributions to cross-cultural psychology* (pp. 88–103). Swets & Zeitlinger.

Hoffman, L. (2019a, May). *An existential-humanistic approach to case conceptualization and treatment planning: Rationale, approach, and limitations* [Paper presentation]. The Second World Congress of Existential Therapy, Buenos Aires, Argentina.

Hoffman, L. (2019b). Gordo's ghost: An introduction to existential-humanistic perspectives on myth. In L. Hoffman, M. Yang, F. J. Kaklauskas, A. Chan, & M. Mansilla (Eds.), *Existential psychology East-West* (Vol. 1, Rev. & expanded ed., pp. 273–288). University Professors Press.

Hoffman, L. (2019c). Introduction to existential-humanistic psychology in a cross-cultural context. In L. Hoffman, M. Yang, F. J. Kaklauskas, A. Chan, & M. Mansilla (Eds.), *Existential psychology East-West* (Vol. 1, Rev. & expanded ed., pp. 1–72). University Professors Press.

Hoffman, L. (2020). Culture and empathy in humanistic psychology. In L. Hoffman, H. P. Cleare-Hoffman, N. Granger, Jr., & D. St. John (Eds.), *Humanistic approaches to multiculturalism and diversity: Perspectives on existence and difference* (pp. 103–116). Routledge. https://doi.org/10.4324/9781351133357-9

Hoffman, L. (2021). Existential-humanistic therapy and disaster response: Lessons from the COVID-19 pandemic. *Journal of Humanistic Psychology, 61*(1), 33–54. https://doi.org/10.1177/0022167820931987

Hoffman, L. (2024). The possibilities and the slippery slope of evidence-based practice in psychology: Why humanistic and existential psychologists must engage the conversation. *The Humanistic Psychologist, 52*(3), 318–324. https://doi.org/10.1037/hum0000347

Hoffman, L. (2025). Approaching existential–humanistic psychotherapy from an evidence-based perspective. In L. Hoffman & V. Lac (Eds.), *The evidence-based foundations of existential–humanistic therapy* (pp. 11–38). American Psychological Association. https://doi.org/10.1037/0000446-002

Hoffman, L., & Cleare-Hoffman, H. P. (2017a, August 3–6). *An existential-humanistic approach to case formulation and treatment planning* [Poster presentation]. American Psychological Association 125th Annual Conference, Washington, DC, United States.

Hoffman, L., & Cleare-Hoffman, H. P. (2017b, October 6–8). *Existential-humanistic case conceptualization and treatment planning with diverse populations: Ethical considerations and adaptations* [Paper presentation]. International Society for Ethical Psychology and Psychiatry 20th Annual Conference, Denver, CO, United States.

Hoffman, L., & Cleare-Hoffman, H. P. (2018a, March 22–25). *Applications of existential-humanistic case conceptualization and treatment planning* [Paper presentation]. Society for Humanistic Psychology 11th Annual Conference, Boulder, CO, United States.

Hoffman, L., & Cleare-Hoffman, H. P. (2018b, August 9–12). Researching existential-humanistic case conceptualization and treatment planning. In L. Hoffman (Chair), *Existential-humanistic case conceptualization and treatment planning* [Symposium]. American Psychological Association 126th Annual Conference, San Francisco, CA, United States.

Hoffman, L., & Islam, S. (2026). Relationality, isolation, and alienation. In L. Hoffman (Ed.), *APA handbook of humanistic and existential psychology* (Vol. 1, pp. 495–520). American Psychological Association. https://doi.org/10.1037/0000431-021

Hoffman, L., & Lac, V. (Eds.). (2025). *The evidence-based foundations of existential–humanistic therapy*. American Psychological Association. https://doi.org/10.1037/0000446-000

Hoffman, L., Lopez, A., & Moats, M. (2013). Humanistic psychology and self-acceptance. In M. Bernard (Ed.), *The strength of self-acceptance: Theory, research, and practice* (pp. 3–17). Springer. https://doi.org/10.1007/978-1-4614-6806-6_1

Hoffman, L., Ramey, B., & Silveira, D. (2020). Existential therapy, religion, and mindfulness. In K. Vail & C. Routledge (Eds.), *The science of religion, spirituality, and existentialism* (pp. 359–369). Elsevier. https://doi.org/10.1016/B978-0-12-817204-9.00026-3

Hoffman, L., Stewart, S., Warren, D., & Meek, L. (2009). Toward a sustainable myth of self: An existential response to the postmodern condition. *Journal of Humanistic Psychology, 49*(2), 135–173. https://doi.org/10.1177/0022167808324880

Hoffman, L., & Vallejos, L. (2018). Existential shattering. In D. Leeming (Ed.), *The encyclopedia of psychology and religion* (3rd ed., pp. 847–850). Springer.

Hoffman, L., Vallejos, L., Cleare-Hoffman, H. P., & Rubin, S. (2015). Emotion, relationship, and meaning as core existential practice: Evidence-based foundations. *Journal of Contemporary Psychotherapy, 45*(1), 11–20. https://doi.org/10.1007/s10879-014-9277-9

Hoffman, L., Yang, M., Kaklauskas, F. J., Chan, A., & Mansilla, M. (Eds.). (2019). *Existential psychology East-West* (Vol. 1, Rev. & expanded ed.). University Professors Press.

Hoffman, L., Yang, M., Mansilla, M., Dias, J., Moats, M., & Claypool, T. (Eds.). (2019). *Existential psychology East-West* (Vol. 2). University Professors Press.

Howard, K. I., Kopta, S. M., Krause, M. S., & Orlinsky, D. E. (1986). The dose–effect relationship in psychotherapy. *American Psychologist, 41*(2), 159–164. https://doi.org/10.1037/0003-066X.41.2.159

Ingle, M. (2026). Rethinking individualism, collectivism, and conformity. In L. Hoffman (Ed.), *APA handbook of humanistic and existential psychology* (Vol. 1, pp. 565–584). American Psychological Association. https://doi.org/10.1037/0000431-024

Jackson, T. (2020). The history of Black psychology and humanistic psychology. In L. Hoffman, H. P. Cleare-Hoffman, N. Granger, Jr., & D. St. John (Eds.), *Humanistic approaches to multiculturalism and diversity: Perspectives on existence and difference* (pp. 29–44). Routledge.

Jackson, T. R., & Pintauro, M. E. (2026). Existential–humanistic psychology's rightful place in the trauma discourse. In L. Hoffman (Ed.), *APA handbook of humanistic and existential psychology* (Vol. 2, pp. 229–244). American Psychological Association. https://doi.org/10.1037/0000432-011

Johnstone, L. (2018). Psychological formulation as an alternative to psychiatric diagnosis. *Journal of Humanistic Psychology, 58*(1), 30–46. https://doi.org/10.1177/0022167817722230

Johnstone, L. (2022). General patterns in the power threat meaning framework: Principles and practice. *Journal of Constructivist Psychology, 35*(1), 16–26. https://doi.org/10.1080/10720537.2020.1773358

Johnstone, L., & Boyle, M. (2018). The power threat meaning framework: An alternative nondiagnostic conceptual system. *Journal of Humanistic Psychology.* Advance online publication. https://doi.org/10.1177/0022167818793289

Jones, W. H. (1982). Loneliness and social behavior. In L. A. Peplau & D. Perlman (Eds.), *Loneliness: A sourcebook of current theory, research, and therapy* (pp. 238–252). Wiley-Interscience.

Jongsma, A. E., Jr., Peterson, L. M., & Bruce, T. J. (2021). *The complete adult psychotherapy treatment planner* (6th ed.). Wiley.

Kamens, S. R., Cosgrove, L., Peters, S. M., Jones, N., Flanagan, E., Longden, E., Schulz, S., Robbins, B. D., Olsen, S., Miller, R., & Lichtenberg, P. (2019). Standards and guidelines for the development of diagnostic nomenclatures and alternatives in mental health research and practice. *Journal of Humanistic Psychology*, *59*(3), 401–427. https://doi.org/10.1177/0022167818763862

Kamens, S. R., Elkins, D. N., & Robbins, B. D. (2017). Open letter to the *DSM-5*. *Journal of Humanistic Psychology*, *57*(6), 675–687. https://doi.org/10.1177/0022167817698261

Kamens, S. R., Flanagan, E. H., & Robbins, B. D. (2018). Introduction to the second special issue on diagnostic alternatives. *Journal of Humanistic Psychology*, *58*(1), 3–6. https://doi.org/10.1177/0022167817718709

Kamens, S. R., Flanagan, E. H., & Robbins, B. D. (2019). Introduction to the fourth special issue on diagnostic alternatives. *Journal of Humanistic Psychology*, *59*(3), 315–318. https://doi.org/10.1177/0022167818787966

Kamens, S. R., Robbins, B. D., & Flanagan, E. H. (2017). Introduction to the special issues on diagnostic alternatives. *Journal of Humanistic Psychology*, *57*(6), 567–572. https://doi.org/10.1177/0022167817701253

Kamens, S. R., Robbins, B. D., & Flanagan, E. H. (2019a). Introduction to the third special issue on diagnostic alternatives. *Journal of Humanistic Psychology*, *59*(1), 3–5. https://doi.org/10.1177/0022167818787963

Kamens, S. R., Robbins, B. D., & Flanagan, E. H. (2019b). Introduction to the fifth special issue on diagnostic alternatives. *Journal of Humanistic Psychology*. Advance online publication. https://doi.org/10.1177/0022167819884135

Karter, J. M., & Kamens, S. R. (2019). Toward conceptual competence in psychiatric diagnosis: An ecological model for critiques of the *DSM*. In S. Steingard (Ed.), *Critical psychiatry: Controversies and clinical implications* (pp. 17–69). Springer. https://doi.org/10.1007/978-3-030-02732-2_2

Kolden, G. G., Wang, C.-C., Austin, S. B., Chang, Y., & Klein, M. H. (2018). Congruence/genuineness: A meta-analysis. *Psychotherapy*, *55*(4), 424–433. https://doi.org/10.1037/pst0000162

Krippner, S. (1990). Personal mythology: An introduction to the concept. *The Humanistic Psychologist*, *18*(2), 137–142. https://doi.org/10.1080/08873267.1990.9976884

Kriz, J., & Längle, A. (2012). A European perspective on the position papers. *Psychotherapy*, *49*(4), 475–479. https://doi.org/10.1037/a0028027

Krug, O. T. (2009). James Bugental and Irvin Yalom: Two masters of existential therapy cultivate presence in the therapeutic encounter. *Journal of Humanistic Psychology*, *49*(3), 329–354. https://doi.org/10.1177/0022167809334001

Krug, O. T. (2019). Existential-humanistic and existential-integrative therapy: Method and practice. In E. van Durzen, E. Craig, A. Längle, K. J. Schneider, D. Tantam, & S. du Pluck (Eds.), *The Wiley world handbook of existential therapy* (pp. 257–266). Wiley. https://doi.org/10.1002/9781119167198.ch15

Krug, O. T., Bradshaw, C., Ratner, J., & Sánchez-Mazarro, A. (2025). Therapeutic presence in existential–humanistic therapy. In L. Hoffman & V. Lac (Eds.), *The evidence-based foundations of existential–humanistic therapy* (pp. 103–130). American Psychological Association. https://doi.org/10.1037/0000446-005

Krug, O. T., & Schneider, K. J. (2016). *Supervision essentials for existential–humanistic therapy*. American Psychological Association. https://doi.org/10.1037/14951-000

Laing, R. D. (1969). *The divided self*. Random House.

Lambert, M. J., & Archer, A. (2006). Research findings on the effects of psychotherapy and their implications for practice. In C. D. Goodheart, A. E. Kazdin, & R. J. Sternberg (Eds.), *Evidence-based psychotherapy: Where practice and research meet* (pp. 111–130). American Psychological Association. https://doi.org/10.1037/11423-005

Levy, K. N., & Anderson, T. (2013). Is clinical psychology doctoral training becoming less intellectually diverse? And if so, what can be done? *Clinical Psychology, 20*(2), 211–220. https://doi.org/10.1111/cpsp.12035

Lewis, G. (1995). *Fanon and the crisis of European man: An essay on philosophy and the human sciences*. Routledge.

Lingiardi, V., & McWilliams, N. (Eds.). (2017). *Psychodynamic diagnostic manual* (2nd ed.). Guilford Press.

Mahendran, D. (2022). The facticity of blackness: A non-conceptual approach to the study of race and racism in Fanon's and Merleau-Ponty's phenomenology. In L. Laubscher, D. Hook, & M. U. Desai (Eds.), *Fanon, phenomenology, and psychology* (pp. 138–150). Routledge.

May, R. (1958). Contributions of existential psychotherapy. In R. May, E. Angel, & H. F. Ellenberger (Eds.), *Existence* (pp. 37–91). Jason Aronson.

May, R. (1969). *Love and will*. Delta.

May, R. (1970). *The meaning of anxiety*. Norton. (Original work published 1950)

May, R. (1981). *Freedom and responsibility*. Norton.

May, R. (1991). *The cry for myth*. Delta.

Mayers, A. M., Khoo, S. T., & Svartberg, M. (2002). The Existential Loneliness Questionnaire: Background, development, and preliminary findings. *Journal of Clinical Psychology, 58*(9), 1183–1193. https://doi.org/10.1002/jclp.10038

Mearns, D., & Cooper, M. (2017). *Working at relational depth in counseling and psychotherapy* (2nd ed.). Sage.

Mendelowitz, E. (2008). *Ethics and Lao Tzu: Intimations of character*. University of the Rockies Press.

Morrill, Z. (2025). Genuineness and the real relationship in existential–humanistic psychotherapy. In L. Hoffman & V. Lac (Eds.), *The evidence-based foundations of existential–humanistic therapy* (pp. 267–292). American Psychological Association. https://doi.org/10.1037/0000446-012

Mosig, Y. D. (2006). Conceptions of the self in Western and Eastern psychology. *Journal of Theoretical and Philosophical Psychology, 26*(1–2), 39–50. https://doi.org/10.1037/h0091266

Norcross, J. C., & Wampold, B. E. (2019). Evidence-based psychotherapy responsiveness: The third task force. In J. C. Norcross & B. E. Wampold (Eds.), *Psychotherapy relationships that work* (Vol. 2, pp. 1–14). Oxford University Press.

O'Donohue, J. (1998). *Anam cara: A Celtic book of Wisdom*. Harper Collins.

Pavlo, A. J. (2026). "A little stand-offish": Existential and humanistic diagnostic perspectives. In L. Hoffman (Ed.), *APA handbook of humanistic and existential psychology* (Vol. 1, pp. 349–364). American Psychological Association. https://doi.org/10.1037/0000431-015

Pavlo, A. J., Flanagan, E. H., Leitner, L. M., & Davidson, L. (2019). Can there be a recovery-oriented diagnostic practice? *The Journal of Humanistic Psychology, 59*(3), 319–338. https://doi.org/10.1177/0022167818787609

Pyszczynski, T., & Diarra, M. (2026). Terror management theory: Toward a merger of existential and experimental approaches to understanding human behavior and experience. In L. Hoffman (Ed.), *APA handbook of humanistic and existential psychology* (Vol. 1, pp. 405–430). American Psychological Association. https://doi.org/10.1037/0000431-017

Robbins, B. D. (2018). *The medicalized body and anesthetic culture: The cadaver, the memorial body, and the recovery of lived experience.* Palgrave.

Robbins, B. D. (2023). The erotic in anesthetic culture: Revisiting Rollo May's concept of "the new puritanism." In S. Simpson, M. Racho, B. D. Robbins, & L. Hoffman (Eds.), *Eros & psyche: Existential perspectives on sexuality* (Vol. 1, pp. 50–89). University Professors Press.

Robbins, B. D., Kamens, S. R., & Elkins, D. N. (2017). *DSM-5* reform efforts by the Society for Humanistic Psychology. *Journal of Humanistic Psychology, 57*(6), 602–624. https://doi.org/10.1177/0022167817698617

Rogers, C. R. (1959). A theory of therapy, personality, and interpersonal relationships, as developed in the client-centered framework. In S. Koch (Ed.), *Psychology: A study of science* (Vol. 3, pp. 184–256). McGraw-Hill.

Rogers, C. R. (1980). *A way of being.* Houghton Mifflin.

Saldaña, J. (2016). *The coding manual for qualitative researchers* (3rd ed.). Sage.

Sartre, J. P. (2021). *Being and nothingness.* Washington Square Press. (Original work published 1943)

Schneider, K. J. (1998). Existential processes. In L. S. Greenberg, J. C. Watson, & G. Lietaer (Eds.), *Handbook of experiential psychotherapy* (pp. 103–120). Guilford Press.

Schneider, K. J. (2004). *Rediscovery of awe: Splendor, mystery, and the fluid center of life.* Paragon House.

Schneider, K. J. (2007). *Existential-integrative psychotherapy: Guideposts to the core of practice.* Routledge.

Schneider, K. J. (2009). *Awakening to awe: Personal stories of profound transformation.* Jason Aronson.

Schneider, K. J. (2013). *The polarized mind: Why it's killing us and what we can do about it.* University Professors Press.

Schneider, K. J. (2015). Presence: The core contextual factor of effective psychotherapy. *Existential Analysis, 2*(2), 304–312.

Schneider, K. J. (2019a). Existential-humanistic and existential-integrative therapy: Philosophy and theory. In E. van Durzen, E. Craig, A. Längle, K. J. Schneider, D. Tantam, & S. du Pluck (Eds.), *The Wiley world handbook of existential therapy* (pp. 247–256). Wiley. https://doi.org/10.1002/9781119167198.ch14

Schneider, K. J. (2019b). *The spirituality of awe: Challenges to the robotic revolution* (2nd ed.). University Professors Press.

Schneider, K. J. (2023). *Life-enhancing anxiety: Key to a sane world.* University Professors Press.

Schneider, K. J., & Hoffman, L. (2024). Existential-humanistic and existential-integrative theory. In F. T. L. Leong, J. L. Callahan, J. Zimmerman, M. J. Constantino, & C. F. Eubanks (Eds.), *APA handbook of psychotherapy: Theory-driven practice and disorder-driven practice* (pp. 53–69). American Psychological Association. https://doi.org/10.1037/0000353-004

Schneider, K. J., Jackson, T., & Hoffman, L. (in press). Existential-humanistic psychotherapy: An integrative, multicultural perspective. In K. Vail, D. Van Tongeren, B. Schegel, J. Greenberg, L. King, & R. Ryan (Eds.), *Handbook of the science of existential psychology.*

Schneider, K. J., & Krug, O. T. (2017). *Existential–humanistic therapy* (2nd ed.). American Psychological Association. https://doi.org/10.1037/0000042-000

Schneider, K. J., & Krug, O. T. (2026). *Existential–humanistic therapy* (3rd ed.). American Psychological Association. https://doi.org/10.1037/0000463-000

Sease, T. B., Cox, C. R., & Knight, K. (2022). Existential isolation and well-being in justice-involved populations. *Frontiers in Psychology, 13*, Article 1092313. Advance online publication. https://doi.org/10.3389/fpsyg.2022.1092313

Sebree, D., Jr., & Brown, V. (2025). Therapist self-disclosure in existential–humanistic psychotherapy. In L. Hoffman & V. Lac (Eds.), *The evidence-based foundations of existential–humanistic therapy* (pp. 293–310). American Psychological Association. https://doi.org/10.1037/0000446-013

Seely, M. R. (2007). Psychological debriefing may not be clinically effective: Implications for a humanistic approach to trauma intervention. *The Journal of Humanistic Counseling, Education and Development, 46*(2), 172–182. https://doi.org/10.1002/j.2161-1939.2007.tb00034.x

Serlin, I. A., Ho, R. T. H., Kurter Musnitksy, F., & Kennedy, J. R. (2025). The creative and expressive arts therapies and existential–humanistic psychotherapy. In L. Hoffman & V. Lac (Eds.), *The evidence-based foundations of existential–humanistic therapy* (pp. 359–380). American Psychological Association. https://doi.org/10.1037/0000446-016

Shedler, J. (2010). The efficacy of psychodynamic psychotherapy. *American Psychologist, 65*(2), 98–109. https://doi.org/10.1037/a0018378

Spaeth, D., Vanderhoff, J. A., Pintauro, M., & Hoffman, L. (2025). Authenticity, self-awareness, and facing life directly in existential–humanistic psychotherapy. In L. Hoffman & V. Lac (Eds.), *The evidence-based foundations of existential–humanistic therapy* (pp. 183–206). American Psychological Association. https://doi.org/10.1037/0000446-008

Stark, M. (2000). *Modes of therapeutic action*. Jason Aronson.

Sutton, A. (2016). Measuring the effects of self-awareness: Construction of the Self-Awareness Outcomes Questionnaire. *Europe's Journal of Psychology, 12*(4), 645–658. https://doi.org/10.5964/ejop.v12i4.1178

Underwood, J. J. (2025). Here-and-now work in existential–humanistic psychotherapy. In L. Hoffman & V. Lac (Eds.), *The evidence-based foundations of existential–humanistic therapy* (pp. 207–224). American Psychological Association. https://doi.org/10.1037/0000446-009

Vallejos, L., & Johnson, Z. (2020). Multicultural competencies in humanistic psychology. In L. Hoffman, H. P. Cleare Hoffman, N. Granger, Jr., & D. St. John (Eds.), *Humanistic approaches to multiculturalism and diversity: Perspectives on existence and difference* (pp. 63–75). Routledge.

van Deurzen, E. (2026). Contemporary considerations of freedom. In L. Hoffman (Ed.), *APA handbook of humanistic and existential psychology* (Vol. 1, pp. 431–448). American Psychological Association. https://doi.org/10.1037/0000431-018

van Deurzen, E., Craig, E., Längle, A., Schneider, K. J., Tantam, D., & du Plock, S. (Eds.). (2019). *The Wiley world handbook of existential therapy*. Wiley. https://doi.org/10.1002/9781119167198

van Deurzen, E., & Kenward, R. (2005). *Dictionary of existential psychotherapy and counseling*. Sage.

Varisco, B., & Hoffman, L. (2025). Working with emotions in existential–humanistic psychotherapy. In L. Hoffman & V. Lac (Eds.), *The evidence-based foundations of existential–humanistic therapy* (pp. 157–182). American Psychological Association. https://doi.org/10.1037/0000446-007

Vincent, A., & Lac, V. (2025). An existential–humanistic approach to equine-facilitated psychotherapy. In L. Hoffman & V. Lac (Eds.), *The evidence-based foundations of existential–humanistic therapy* (pp. 397–412). American Psychological Association. https://doi.org/10.1037/0000446-018

Vos, J. (2018). *Meaning in life: An evidence-based handbook for practitioners*. Red Globe Press.

Vos, J. (2025a). Existential–therapeutic competencies. In L. Hoffman & V. Lac (Eds.), *The evidence-based foundations of existential–humanistic therapy* (pp. 39–68). American Psychological Association. https://doi.org/10.1037/0000446-003

Vos, J. (2025b). Working with meaning in life in existential–humanistic psychotherapy. In L. Hoffman & V. Lac (Eds.), *The evidence-based foundations of existential–humanistic therapy* (pp. 225–252). American Psychological Association. https://doi.org/10.1037/0000446-010

Vos, J. (2026). Meaning in life and society. In L. Hoffman (Ed.), *APA handbook of humanistic and existential psychology* (Vol. 2, pp. 501–534). American Psychological Association. https://doi.org/10.1037/0000432-025

Vos, J., & Vitali, D. (2018). The effects of psychological meaning-centered therapies on quality of life and psychological stress: A metaanalysis. *Palliative & Supportive Care, 16*(5), 608–632. https://doi.org/10.1017/S1478951517000931

Wampold, B. E. (2008, February 4). Existential-integrative psychotherapy: Coming of age [Review of the book *Existential-integrative psychotherapy: Guideposts to the core of practice* by K. J. Schneider]. *APA PsycCRITIQUES, 53*(6). https://doi.org/10.1037/a0011070

Wampold, B. E., & Imel, Z. E. (2015). *The great psychotherapy debate: Models, methods, findings* (2nd ed.). Routledge. https://doi.org/10.4324/9780203582015

Wang, X. (2019). The symbol of the iron house: From survivalism to existentialism. In L. Hoffman, M. Yang, M. Mansilla, J. Dias, M. Moats, & T. Claypool (Eds.), *Existential psychology East-West* (Vol. 2, pp. 3–16). University Professors Press.

Watson, J. C., Greenberg, L. S., & Lietaer, G. (1998). The experiential paradigm unfolding: Relationship and experiencing in therapy. In L. S. Greenberg, J. C. Watson, & G. Lietaer (Eds.), *Handbook of experiential psychotherapy* (pp. 3–27). Guilford Press.

Whaley, A. L. (2011). Clinicians' competence in assessing cultural mistrust among African American psychiatric patients. *The Journal of Black Psychology, 37*(4), 387–406. https://doi.org/10.1177/0095798410387133

Wickramasekera, I. E., II. (2007). Empathic features of absorption and incongruence. *The American Journal of Clinical Hypnosis, 50*(1), 59–69. https://doi.org/10.1080/00029157.2007.10401598

Wolfe, B. E. (2008). Existential issues in anxiety disorders and their treatment. In K. J. Schneider (Ed.), *Existential-integrative psychotherapy: Guideposts to the core of practice* (pp. 204–216). Routledge.

Wong, P. T. P. (2012). Toward a dual-systems model of what makes life worth living. In P. T. P. Wong (Ed.), *Meaning: Theories, research, and applications* (2nd ed.). Taylor & Francis.

Wood, A. (2005). Alienation. In T. Honderich (Ed.), *The Oxford companion to philosophy* (p. 21). Oxford University Press.

World Health Organization. (2019). *International statistical classification of diseases and related health problems* (11th ed.). https://icd.who.int/

Yalom, I. D. (1980). *Existential psychotherapy*. Basic Books.

Yalom, I. D. (2013). *The gift of therapy: An open letter to a new generation of therapists and their patients*. Harper Perennial.

Yang, M. (2020). *Lighting the candle: Taoist principles in supervision conducted from an existential-humanistic perspective*. University Professors Press.

INDEX

A

Abbreviated process, of EH case formulation, 36–37
Acceptance, 58
Agency, 123–127
Alienation, 127–135
Alternative diagnosis, 103
American Psychological Association (APA)
    APA Dictionary of Psychology, 124
    Presidential Task Force on Evidence-Based Practice, 163
American Psychologist, 157
Anticipated challenges, 152–153
Anxiety, life-enhancing, 52
APA Dictionary of Psychology (American Psychological Association), 124
Approaches, to case formulations, 14
Authenticity, 53–54

B

Bad faith, 124
Bahamas, 133
Baldwin, J., 125
Barriers, anticipated, 152–153
Beauvoir, S. de, 53, 107, 125
Becker, E., 120–121
Bias, cultural, 10
Biological and physical considerations, 108–109
Black individuals, 10
Black Skin, White Masks (Fanon), 9
Blind spots, cultural, 9

Bohart, A. C., 88, 90, 151
Brief holistic client narrative, 87–91
    Hank (case example), 170–171
    Jacinta (case example), 192
    Rasheeda (case example), 90–91
Brown, V., 57–58
Buddhism, 60
Bugental, J. F. T., 6, 44, 53, 119–120

C

Camus, A., 124
Case formulation
    approaches to, 6–7, 14
    colonization of, 7–11
    future directions, for research, 206
    as guide for EH therapy, 37–38
    techniques of, 14
    template for, 28–30, 207–217
CBT (cognitive behavior therapy), 8
Challenges, anticipated, 152–153
China, 6, 8–9
Clarification, of presenting concerns and focus, 23–26
Cleare-Hoffman, H. P., 133
Client goals, initial, 150–151
Client's description of the concern or problem, 95–98
Client strengths and resources, 107–108
Client–therapist relationship, 143–145
Cognitive behavior therapy (CBT), 8
Colonization, of case conceptualization, 7–11

The Complete Adult Psychotherapy Treatment Planner (Jongsma), 152
Concern or problem identification
    alternative diagnosis, 29, 103
    client's description of the concern or problem, 95–98
    diagnosis of systems or contextual issues, 98–100
    Hank (case example), 171–173
    ICD-11 or *DSM-5* diagnosis, 102–103
    implications of concern or problem, 99–101
    Jacinta (case example), 193–194
    legal and ethical issues, 101–102
Connecting markers, 23–24
Cooper, M., 6, 34, 44, 50
Craig, Erik, 6
Creative and expressive arts interventions, 60
The Cry for Myth (May), 140
Cultural bias, 10
Cultural blind spots, 9
Cultural considerations, 112–113
Curiosity, 19–20, 52

D

Daimonic, 141–143, 180, 200
Davis, Terri, 6, 144
Death, 120–123
Destiny, 124
Diagnosis, alternative, 103
Diagnosis of systems or contextual issues, 98–100
Diagnostic and Statistical Manual of Mental Disorders (American Psychiatric Association), 10, 102–103
Diamond, S. A., 142
Diarra, M., 120

E

Eels, T. D., 11, 25, 93
EH treatment strategies and interventions, 154
Elkins, D. N., 6, 26
Ellenberger, H. F., 53
Embodied curiosity, 19–20
Embodied empathy, 50
Embodiment, 15–16, 135–138
Emergent client goals, 151–152
Emotions, 21, 50–53, 135–138
Empathy, 16, 50–51
Employment considerations, 111–112
Engaging in therapy, 31
Ethical dimensions of freedom, 126
Ethical issues, 101–102
The Evidence-Based Foundations of Existential–Humanistic Psychotherapy (Hoffman & Lac), 157–159

Evidence-based practice, 157–159, 163
Existential givens, 119–120
Existential–humanistic (EH) interventions, 41–62
    authenticity, self-awareness, and facing life directly, 53–54
    emotional processing, 52–53
    empathy, 50–51
    genuineness and the real relationship, 51–52
    identifying, 42–44
    integrative strategies, 59–61
    meaning-centered interventions, 55–56
    objective or guiding stances and psychoeducation, 58–59
    positive regard or acceptance, 58
    presence, 49–50
    protections and resistance, 54–55
    self-disclosure, 57–58
Existential isolation, 129–130
Existential loneliness, 130–132
Existential Psychotherapy (Yalom), 130
Existential shattering, 54
Experiential techniques, 60
Exploration, continued, 25

F

Facing life directly, 53–54
Family considerations, 109–112
Family dynamics, 8–9
Fanon, F., 9–10, 98, 133
Filial piety, 8–9
Finiteness, 120–123
Framework, for EH case formulation, 13–39
    abbreviated process of, 36–37
    assessing for goodness of fit, 31–33
    connecting markers in, 23–24
    connecting with hope, 33–34
    early sessions, 34–35
    embodied curiosity, 19–20
    embodiment, vs. technique, 15–16
    establishing a good therapeutic relationship and engaging in therapy, 31
    first session, 30–31
    as guide for EH therapy, 37–38
    helping clients clarify presenting concerns and focus, 24–25
    marking patterns and potential concerns, 20–23
    ongoing process of, 35–36
    phenomenological strategies or stances, 16–19
    presence, 15
    timelines, fluidity, and case formulation, 25–28
Frankl, V. E., 6, 53, 55, 126, 139
Freedom, 123–127
Freire, P., 7

G

Gelso, C. J., 51
Genuineness, 51–52
Goals, initial client, 150–151
Goldman, R. N., 94
Goodness of fit, 31–33
Greenberg, L. S., 50, 94
Greening, T., 54, 119, 151
Grounding techniques, 89
Guiding stances, 58–59

H

Hank (case example), 166–184
  brief holistic client narrative, 170–171
  concern or problem identification,
    171–173
  introduction to, 166–169
  sessions 9 to 30, 169–170
  theoretical aspects of the case formulation,
    173–181
  treatment planning, 181–184
Heery, Myrtle, 6
Here-and-now, 22, 56–57, 117–118
Historical-racial schema, 10
Hocoy, D., 133
Hoffman, L., 6, 133, 157–159
Hope, connecting with, 33–34
How Clients Make Therapy Work (Bohart
    & Tallman), 88

I

ICD-11 (*International Classification of
    Diseases*; World Health Organization),
    102–103
Identifying EH interventions, 42–44
Immediacy. *See* here-and-now
Implications of concern or problem, 99–101
Initial client goals, 150–151
Insurance coverage, 26–27
Integrative strategies, 59–61, 154–155
Interconnectedness of freedom, 125–126
International Classification of Diseases (*ICD-11*;
    World Health Organization), 102–103
International Institute of Existential–
    Humanistic Therapy (China), 6
Interpersonal isolation, 128–129
Interpretative markers, 22
Interventions, 42
  creative and expressive arts, 60
  existential–humanistic. *See* Existential–
    humanistic (EH) interventions
  meaning-centered, 55–56
  treatment strategies and, 153–154
Intrapersonal isolation, 127–128
Islam, S., 6, 133
Isolation, 127–135

J

Jacinta (case example), 184–204
  brief holistic client narrative, 192
  concern or problem identification,
    193–194
  introduction to, 184–185
  sessions 1 to 8, 185–188
  sessions 9 to 30, 188–192
  theoretical aspects of the case formulation,
    194–201
  treatment planning, 202–204
Jackson, T., 10, 98
Johnstone, L., 13
Jongsma, A. E., Jr., 152
Junkanoo (Bahamian festival), 133

K

Kenward, R., 124
Krippner, S., 140
Krug, O. T., 6, 14, 21, 115

L

Lac, V., 157–159
Laing, R. D., 6
Language, 25
Legal issues, 101–102
Lewis, G., 123
Liberatory potential, 9
Life, facing directly, 53–54
Lingiardi, V., 98
Loneliness, 129–132

M

Mahendran, D., 10
Marking, 20–24
May, R., 6, 19, 44, 52, 123–126, 132,
    140–142
McWilliams, N., 98
Meaning, 139–141
Meaning-centered interventions, 55–56
Mearns, D., 34, 44, 50
Meursault (fictional character), 124
Mindfulness, 60–61
Morrill, Z., 51
Motivation, 115–117
Multicultural issues, 18

N

Narrative of the client's desired outcome,
    28, 149–150
Nonverbal markers, 22
Normal reactions to abnormal situations,
    98, 113
Noting, 20

O

Objective stances, 58–59
Ongoing process, EH case formulation, 35–36

P

Patience, 25
Pattern markers, 22
Pattern seeking, 25
Perls, Fritz, 6
Personal disclosures, 57
Perspective on concern or problem, 97–98
Phenomenological methods, 7
Piety, filial, 8–9
Pink Floyd, 88
Positive regard, 58
Presenting concerns and focus, 23–26
Process markers, 22
Protections, 54–55
Psychodynamic Diagnostic Manual (Lingiardi & McWilliams), 98
Psychoeducation, 58–59
Psychotherapy Case Formulation (Eels), 11
Pyszczynski, T., 120

R

Racism, 9–11, 100, 111–114, 126–127, 133–134, 142, 153
Randomized clinical trials (RCTs), 158–159
Rasheeda (case example), 63–86
    anticipated challenges and/or barriers, 152–153
    biological and physical considerations, 108–109
    brief holistic client narrative, 90–91
    building the therapeutic alliance, developing curiosity, and facilitating emotional processing, 69–73
    client's perspective on concern or problem, 97–98
    client strengths and resources, 107–108
    client–therapist relationship, 144–145
    continued emotional exploration, self-empowerment, and social connection, 83
    cultural considerations, 112–113
    daimonic, 142
    death and finiteness, 122–123
    deepening the therapeutic process, 73, 74–75
    diagnosis of systems or contextual issues, 100
    EH treatment strategies and interventions, 154
    emergent client goals, 152
    emotions and embodiment, 136–138

    engaging and staying with emotions and deepening self-awareness, 74
    family and social considerations, 109–111
    freedom, responsibility and agency, 126–127
    getting to know each other and assessing goodness of fit, 67–69
    here-and-now, 117–118
    ICD-11 or *DSM-5* diagnosis, 102–103
    identifying, disclosing, and processing a sexual assault, 78–83
    implications of concern or problem, 101
    initial client goals, 151
    integrative strategies, 155
    introduction, 64–67
    legal and ethical issues, 102
    meaning, 140–141
    narrative of the client's desired outcome, 149–150
    perspective on concern or problem, 97–98
    processing a sudden, difficult emotional experience, 74–75
    processing grief and feelings of loneliness and isolation, 76–78
    relationships, isolation, and alienation, 134–135
    school and employment considerations, 111–112
    self-acceptance, 143
    self-awareness and motivation, 116–117
    support for treatment approaches, stances, and/or techniques, 160–162
    systemic issues, 113–114
    treatment progress, 155–156
RCTs (randomized clinical trials), 158–159
Real relationships, 51–52
Reasons for entering therapy, 23–26
Reflection of marker themes or patterns, 22
Relationships, 51–52, 127–135
Required initial history gathering and assessment session, 37
Research
    demonstrating support for, 159–162
    future directions for, 206
    on identifying E-H interventions, 42–43
Resistance, 54–55
Responsibility, 123–127
Robbins, B. D., 132
Rogers, C. R., 6, 15, 50
Role of theory, in EH psychotherapy, 17–19

S

Saldaña, J., 23
Sartre, J. P., 53
Schneider, K. J., 6, 14–15, 21, 44, 49–50, 54–56, 120
School considerations, 111–112

Sease, T. B., 131
Sebree, D., Jr., 57–58
Seely, M. R., 88–89
Self-acceptance, 142–143
Self-awareness, 53–54, 115–117
Self-disclosure, 57–58
Sexism, 100, 111, 114, 126, 134, 142,
    153, 156
Shattering, existential, 54
Shortened timeline, for report, 37
Significant event markers, 21
Silberberg, A., 51
Silent markers, 22
Social considerations, 109–112
Stances
    as basis for EH therapy, 14
    embodied curiosity, 19–20
    embodiment, vs. technique, 15–16
    objective, 58–59
    phenomenology, 16–19
    presence, 15, 49–50
    support for, 160–162
Sterling, M. M., 119
The Stranger (Camus), 124
Strategies, phenomenological, 16–19
Support for treatment approaches, stances,
    and/or techniques, 157–163
    demonstrating research support,
        159–162
    evidence-based practice, 157–159
Synthesis, of (EH), 46–49
Systemic issues, 113–114

T

Tagging, 20
Tallman, K., 88
Technique, vs. embodiment, 15–16
Techniques, of case formulation, 14
Techniques, support for, 160–162
Template, for EH case formulation, 207–217
Terror management theory (TMT),
    120–121
Theme markers, 22
Theoretical aspects of case formulation, 29
    client strengths and resources, 107–108
    client–therapist relationship, 143–145
    cultural considerations, 112–113
    daimonic, 141–142
    death and finiteness, 120–123
    emotions and embodiment, 135–138
    existential givens, 119–120
    family and social considerations, 109–112
    freedom, responsibility and agency,
        123–127
    Hank (case example), 173–181

here-and-now, 117–118
    Jacinta (case example), 194–201
    meaning, 139–141
    relationships, isolation, and alienation,
        127–135
    self-acceptance, 142–143
    self-awareness and motivation, 115–117
    systemic issues, 113–114
Therapeutic relationship, establishing, 31
Therapist's participation, in emotion, 50–51
Therapy relationship markers, 22
TMT (terror management theory), 120–121
Transference process, 7–8
Treatment approaches, support for,
    160–162
Treatment goals, 152
Treatment planning, 29–30, 147–156
    anticipated challenges and/or barriers,
        152–153
    EH treatment strategies and interventions,
        153–154
    emergent client goals, 151–152
    Hank (case example), 181–184
    initial client goals, 150–151
    integrative strategies, 154–155
    Jacinta (case example), 202–204
    narrative of the client's desired outcome,
        149–150
    treatment goals, 152
    treatment progress, 155–156
Treatment progress, 155–156
Treatment strategies and interventions,
    153–154

V

Van Deurzen, E., 124, 126
Vitali, D., 55
Vocalized markers, 22
Voicing, 50
Vos, J., 54, 55, 139

W

Wampold, B. E., 14
Wang, X., 54, 139
Watson, J. C., 60
Whaley, A. L., 10
Wickramasekera, I. E., II, 15
Wolfe, B. E., 31
World Health Organization, 102–103

Y

Yalom, I. D., 4, 6, 26, 119, 122, 129–130
Yang, M., 41

ABOUT THE AUTHORS

Louis Hoffman, PhD, is a licensed psychologist in private practice and the executive director of the Rocky Mountain Humanistic Counseling and Psychological Association. An avid writer, Dr. Hoffman has published over 20 books and 100 journal articles and book chapters. His books include the *APA Handbook of Humanistic and Existential Psychology, Eros & Psyche: Existential Perspectives on Sexuality, Existential Psychology East-West* (Volumes 1 & 2), and *Becoming an Existential–Humanistic Therapist*. He has been recognized as a fellow of the American Psychological Association and six of its divisions (1: The Society for General Psychology & Interdisciplinary Inquiry; 10: Society for the Psychology of Aesthetics, Creativity, & the Arts; 32: Society for Humanistic Psychology; 36: Society for Psychology of Religion and Spirituality; 48: Society for the Study of Peace, Conflict and Violence: Peace Psychology Division; & 52: International Psychology) and is a recipient of the Rollo May Award of the Society for Humanistic Psychology. He serves on the editorial boards of the *Journal of Humanistic Psychology* (as senior international editor) and the *Journal of Constructivist Psychology*. He is the incoming editor of *The Humanistic Psychologist* and will assume the full-time editor role in 2026.

Heatherlyn P. Cleare-Hoffman, PsyD, is a staff psychologist at the Gallogly Wellness Center at the University of Colorado at Colorado Springs. She previously served as the associate director for Clinical Training at Argosy University, San Francisco Bay Area; core faculty at the University of the Rockies; and clinical director at the Center for Growth. Originally from the Bahamas, Dr. Cleare-Hoffman studied psychology in the Bahamas, Canada, and the United States before obtaining her psychology degree. She was a keynote speaker at the Society for Humanistic Psychology's 12th Annual Conference in 2019. Dr. Cleare-Hoffman's research interests include multicultural psychology, international psychology, cultural rituals and festivals, and the psychological implications of Junkanoo for Bahamians. She is coeditor of *Humanistic Approaches to Multiculturalism and Diversity: Perspectives on Existence and Difference.*